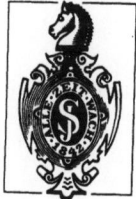

Peter I. Folb

The Safety of Medicines
Evaluation and Prediction

Foreword by J.R. Trounce

Springer-Verlag
Berlin Heidelberg New York 1980

Peter I. Folb, M.D., F.R.C.P., F.C.P.(S.A.)
Professor of Pharmacology, University of Cape Town;
Chief Physician, Groote Schuur Hospital, Cape Town,
South Africa

ISBN-13:978-3-540-10143-7   e-ISBN-13:978-1-4471-3103-8
DOI: 10.1007/978-1-4471-3103-8

Library of Congress Cataloging in Publication Data. Folb, Peter I. 1938— The safety of medicines, evaluation and prediction. Bibliography: p. Includes index. 1. Drugs—Side effects. 2. Drugs—Safety measures. 3. Drugs—Testing. 4. Drug utilization—Evaluation. I. Title. RM302.5.F64 615'.7'0287 80-17994 ISBN-13:978-3-540-10143-7 (U.S.)

This work is subject to copyright. All rights are reserved, whether the whole or part of the material is concerned, specifically those of translation, reprinting, re-use of illustrations, broadcasting, reproduction by photocopying machine or similar means, and storage in data banks. Under § 54 of the German Copyright Law where copies are made for other than private use, a fee is payable to the publisher, the amount of the fee to be determined by agreement with the publisher.

© by Springer-Verlag Berlin Heidelberg 1980

The use of general descriptive names, trade names, trade marks, etc. in this publication, even if the former are not especially identified, is not to be taken as a sign that such names, as understood by the Trade Marks and Merchandise Marks Act, may accordingly be used freely by anyone.

Typesetting: Photo-Graphics, Stockland, Honiton, Devon, England

2128/3916-54320

To Susan

Foreword

The last thirty years have seen an unprecedented increase in the discovery of new drugs, and moreover, these drugs, unlike many of the nostra of former times, have varied and powerful pharmacological actions.

The occurrence of one or two "drug disasters", together with a change in public attitudes, has made it necessary for governments to introduce legislation to control the introduction and release of new therapeutic agents, and most countries in the Western World have some form of drug licensing agency. Whole series of regulations have appeared which aim at discovering and defining the toxicity of new drugs. Many of these regulations rely heavily on testing drugs in animals before they are used in man, and at present very extensive and prolonged animal studies are required by most licensing authorities.

It is most opportune that Professor Folb has decided to review the present position in this monograph. It is not only inhumane but also wasteful of time and money if extensive animal experiments which have little or no relevance to the human situation are carried out; furthermore, such results may even be dangerously misleading. There is little doubt that some preliminary animal investigations are necessary, but it is essential to keep their relevance under continuous review and to adopt a critical and flexible approach rather than heap regulation upon regulation. Professor Folb has done a most useful service, not only to those concerned with drug regulation and drug usage (including most of the medical profession) but also to the public, who ultimately have much to gain from a clear-sighted and unbiased approach to this difficult subject.

London, 1980
J.R. Trounce M.D., F.R.C.P.
Professor of Clinical Pharmacology,
Guy's Hospital Medical School,
London

Preface

Out of this nettle, danger, we pluck this flower, safety

> William Shakespeare
> *Henry IV*

Safety has always been one of the most important of human concerns. As applied to medicines, evaluation of safety cannot be a static or rigid matter but must be flexible and appropriate to changing circumstances. No medicine can be assumed to be completely safe, and in all cases safety evaluation must be a risk-benefit assessment. It is good medical practice, for example, to use an effective though highly toxic medicine in a life-threatening situation, but in an illness that is inevitably self-limiting the use of a medicine with even an extremely small risk of fatal toxicity is unacceptable. In practice "safety" cannot be considered in isolation from "efficacy" and cannot be defined by inflexible guidelines.

However, certain general principles do seem to emerge in considering drug safety. In attempting to define these I hope to be able to contribute towards the ultimate common goal of the developers of new medicines — the pharmaceutical industry, drug regulatory authorities, medical practitioners and the lay public alike — which is to ensure that valuable medicines are made available for patients as simply, economically and swiftly as is reasonably possible. In particular, unnecessarily tedious, expensive and wasteful (and therefore inhumane) animal experimentation must be avoided.

The word "drug" has assumed a certain connotation today, particularly to the lay public, as being a narcotic or opiate, or a medicine with dependence-producing potential, so to minimise confusion the term "medicine" has been preferred in the text, except when the adjectival form was required, e.g. drug-induced diseases. However, in the chapter referring to dependence, reference was confined to "drug", for obvious reasons.

It strikes me that the overriding principle applicable to registration of new medicines is reasonableness. In this regard I am grateful to my colleagues on the South African Medicines Control Council, Professors Bob Charlton and Deo Botha, whose balanced approach to drug registration has influenced my own thinking. My colleagues Roy Keeton, John Gosling, Pat Thompson, Ed Coetzee, Ashley Robins, Frank Bowey and Stephen Cridland have helped me with valuable suggestions and opinions concerning the text of this book.

The South African Medical Research Council has supported my researches into mechanisms and animal models of drug-induced damage, and this help is gratefully acknowledged.

Throughout the preparation of this book I have received dedicated assistance from Renée Gelbart.

Cape Town, 1980   Peter I. Folb

Contents

page

1. **Animal testing and early studies in humans** 1

   1.1. Introduction 1.2. Animal investigations 1.3. Factors influencing animal data 1.4. Extrapolation of data from animals to man 1.5. Metabolite-mediated toxicity 1.6. Early administration of medicines to man 1.7. Summary and conclusions

2. **Prediction of teratogenic potential of a new medicine** 17

   2.1. Drug utilisation during pregnancy
   2.2. The thalidomide model of drug-induced fetal damage
   2.3. The spectrum of teratogenic effects
   2.4. Prediction of the teratogenic potential of a new medicine 2.5. Decision-taking in practice
   2.6. Summary and conclusions

3. **Prediction of dependence-producing potential of a new drug** 29

   3.1. The features of drug dependence in man 3.2. Clinical profiles of drug dependence 3.3 Profile of a drug likely to produce dependence 3.4. Strategy in evaluation of dependence-potential 3.5. Summary and conclusions

4. **Prediction of carcinogenic potential of a new medicine** 49

   4.1. The risks of drug-induced neoplasia in man
   4.2. Profile of the high-risk medicine 4.3. Animal studies
   4.4. Interpretation of animal data 4.5. In vitro tests
   4.6. Summary and conclusions

5. The prediction of adverse drug interactions 63

5.1. The incidence and spectrum of drug-drug interactions
5.2. Clinically important adverse drug interactions
5.3. Prediction of adverse drug interactions 5.4. Clinical guidelines 5.5. Fixed-ratio combinations 5.6. Potential interactions of single-entity medicines 5.7. Summary and conclusions

6. Monitoring drug safety in clinical practice 83

6.1. Introduction 6.2. The diagnosis of adverse drug reactions in practice 6.3. Physicians' evaluations of adverse drug reactions 6.4. Reporting and monitoring of adverse drug reactions 6.5. Risk-benefit evaluations 6.6 Summary and conclusions

Subject Index 101

1 Animal testing and early studies in humans

1.1. Introduction

Laboratory animals have been used for the prediction of the safety of medicines for more than 150 years, and it has become traditional to expose animals to potentially toxic new medicines before they are administered to humans. In many quarters this is argued as being only ethical and fair. It has been stated from theories of evolution that "rodents should give every bit as valid indications of human reactions as dogs", suggesting that results obtained from simple laboratory mice and rats may be as directly translatable to man as those from more highly developed non-primate animals. In practice, carefully designed and executed animal studies often do provide the investigator with valuable information as to the likely safety profile of new chemical entities in humans. However, it must be said that medicines are designed for sick people, not for healthy animals. There are considerable limitations in extrapolating experimental animal data to man. These studies are often wasteful in numbers, particularly when they are faulty in design. Unnecessary sacrifice of animals is a cause of widespread public concern.

Drug evaluation in animals should give a prediction of the likelihood of efficacy of the new entity as well as a profile of its toxicity which includes a broad indication of the safe dose in humans. Sometimes these objectives are met. Sometimes, however, potentially valuable and possibly safe new chemical entities are discarded unnecessarily because of unacceptable animal toxicity which might not necessarily have relevance to humans, and sometimes animal screening may fail to detect a potential for serious human toxicity. Clearly, certain adverse effects are readily predictable from animal studies and others simply cannot be anticipated. The experimental approach has to be designed to meet the requirements of each new entity, and a rigid approach to the study of the toxicity of a medicine must be avoided at all costs.

1.2. Animal investigations

1.2.1. Lethal dose$_{50}$

The lethal dose$_{50}$ (LD_{50}) expresses the dose of a medicine that causes 50% mortality in the group of animals studied. Groups of 5, 10 or 20 animals are usually studied, using at least three different doses (see Sect. 1.2.4. below). The LD_{50} simply expresses whether or not death occurs and as such it reflects acute toxic potency. The LD_{50} of a particular chemical entity is highly species-specific and may vary up to 1000-fold in different animal species.

The particular value of the determination of the LD_{50} in drug development is that it can be compared with the same parameter for related known substances, and comparison can also be made with the effective dose of the same agent, thus giving an idea of the safety margin. Acceptable levels of human exposure to the new chemical entity are projected, and this may be necessary to prevent catastrophe. The essential limitation of the LD_{50} is that it expresses a numerical value which represents the end-result of toxicity. It does not give important information such as time of death, rate of recovery in non-fatal toxicity, and the nature of the two-phase mortality caused by certain medicines. It gives no idea of sites of action and possible mechanisms of toxicity of medicines, nor does it detect non-lethal toxicity. In short, the LD_{50} fails to correlate mortality with morbidity and fails to reflect latent and persistent toxicity.

The LD_{50} varies according to the absorption, distribution and metabolism of the medicine in the animal species concerned. For these reasons, factors such as species differences, genetic constitution, age, sex, and weight of animals may affect the result. Inter-species differences may be particularly marked. Another difficulty in interpreting LD_{50} data is the poor reproducibility between laboratories, which is common.

Drug regulation authorities and those interested in the *post hoc* evaluation of safety of medicines regard the LD_{50} as of limited value. It is of importance to the developers of new medicines, who need to define guidelines, but parameters such as minimum symptomatic dose, minimum toxic dose, and the approximate maximum tolerated dose are of greater interest. An approximate indication of LD_{50} carried out on a small number of animals is usually sufficient; the sacrifice of more animals for this purpose is unnecessary.

1.2.2. Acute toxicity studies

Acute studies offer a valuable lead to more extensive testing. In addition to the LD_{50} they may give indications of the following:

(i) The absorption of a medicine, if tests are done both intravenously and orally and a comparison is made of the doses required to give the same end-point of toxicity. If the oral and intravenous doses are approximately the same, the medicine can be assumed to be well absorbed from the alimentary canal; if not, it may be that absorption is poor or delayed.

(ii) Measurement of blood and tissue levels after acute administration gives a comparison of acute toxicity between different animal species or between the test species and humans, and a correlation of biological effects with drug concentrations may be made.

Further details of acute toxicity studies are included in Sect. 1.2.4.

1.2.3. Prolonged toxicity studies

For any medicine likely to be administered continuously to humans for periods greater than one week or to be given repeatedly, the safety of prolonged administration must be determined. This is necessary to detect possible damage to any organ which may be sensitive to the adverse effects of the medicine, in which case the minimum amount of the medicine or its metabolite likely to cause damage is determined. Prolonged toxicity testing may also help select the best-tolerated compound from a series of chemically related entities with similar action. The design of prolonged toxicity studies is often based on acute toxicity data.

1.2.4. Experimental details

The following details of design and execution are pertinent to acute and prolonged animal toxicity studies:

(i) Choice of species. In choosing a test species the aim is to select one which may be sensitive to the actions and toxic effects of the medicine under investigation, where the patterns of absorption, distribution, metabolism and elimination of the medicine resemble those in man as closely as possible for the same medicine. Such correlation is uncommon, and at least two and sometimes more different species should be examined. Comparison of different species indicates whether a particular species sensitivity exists.

(ii) Choice and care of animals. It is important that the animals examined are not at the extremes of age, as patterns of drug metabolism and the expression of toxicity may be quite different in very young and very old animals. Careful attention must be paid to conditions of husbandry, and exposure to chemicals such as DDT which may modify drug metabolism must be avoided. Both sexes are studied.

(iii) Route of administration. As far as possible the medicine should be administered to the test animals in the same manner as proposed for humans. Intraperitoneal administration to rodents is regarded as equivalent to intravenous administration, provided the medicine concerned does not induce local changes in the peritoneum, such as fibrosis, which may modify the absorption of subsequent doses. When a medicine is intended for topical or oral administration, detailed study of its systemic toxicity has to be carried out in addition to study of its local effects.

(iv) Dose. The responses of test animals to at least three doses are normally determined: the maximum tolerated dose, which will kill some animals in the test groups; a low dose, which approximates to that proposed for use for therapeutic purposes (allowance having been made for body mass; see Table 1.2.); and an intermediate dose falling between the two. Where possible dose-response relationships are defined.

(v) Formulation. It is essential that toxicity studies are carried out on the precise formulation proposed for administration to humans. Even minor modifications in formulation may change the toxicity of a medicine. Examination of the vehicle or excipient is also critical. (The early disaster caused by the inadvertent use of the fatally nephrotoxic diethylene glycol as a solvent for a sulphonamide and the subsequent confirmation of this toxicity in animals gave a strong impetus to preclinical toxicity testing, and it remains a vivid lesson in the minds of all concerned with drug toxicity.) The toxicity of the inactive components alone and in combination with the active principle under investigation has to be determined.

(vi) Duration of study. Most authorities are agreed that all relevant information from prolonged toxicity studies can probably be gained within 3 to 6 months. Animal toxicity investigations lasting longer than this period of time are rarely justified.

(vii) Number of animals. A few animals subjected to a well-designed experimental plan and carefully observed and examined yield results of greater value than more animals less well examined.

(viii) Type of examinations. The following different examinations are important in the assessment of toxicity:

(a) Routine observations, including daily weight and regular clinical examination for organ dysfunction, particularly the central nervous system (CNS). The CNS observations should include examination of muscle tone and attitude and postural and pupillary reflexes.

(b) Regular full blood count and urine examinations form an integral part of toxicity testing. The routine biochemical tests advocated are blood glucose and serum electrolyte estimations. Other, more specialised biochemical investigations are required when particular aspects of organ sensitivity are being specially scrutinised.

(c) Plasma and tissue concentrations of the parent medicine and its metabolite(s) are estimated when feasible. Poor correlation of organ toxicity with plasma levels of the parent compound suggests either that a metabolite may be exerting the toxic effect or that toxicity has been caused by irreversible binding or by "first hit" damage to the tissues. In the latter case the toxic effect lasts long after the medicine and its active metabolites have disappeared from the blood stream.

(d) All test animals are examined post mortem, and histology of the principal organs is undertaken if specific organ sensitivity is suggested by macroscopic observations or biochemical data. In the future the fields of histochemistry and electron microscopy are likely to be important areas in the development of investigative toxicology.

(e) Reproduction is studied in detail. This includes size and number of litters, weight of newborns, details of malformations, and feticidal cannibalism (common amongst drug-treated animals).

(ix) Local irritancy. It is essential that studies of local irritancy are carried out for new medicines designed for topical application to the skin or mucous membranes, or for administration by intramuscular or intravenous injection. It is usually necessary for separate tests to be carried out on the various components of the formulation. The topical effects of a medicine designed for application to the skin are evaluated on intact and abraded skin: topical irritancy may only manifest itself in certain cases when skin integrity has been damaged.

The vagina of the normal human female of child-bearing age is usually highly acid, whereas the vagina of most animals is usually alkaline. These differences in pH frequently make local studies of bioavailability and toxicity difficult to interpret.

(x) Drug hypersensitivity cannot normally be demonstrated in animals, because in the case of human hypersensitivity reactions there is no discernible relationship between the chemical nature of the medicine and its adverse pharmacological effect. Cross-sensitivity which develops in humans between chemicals sharing similar antigenic structure is almost impossible to anticipate in the experimental situation.

1.3. Factors influencing animal data

Factors which influence the quality and reproducibility, and therefore the relevance of animal-derived data, include the following:

(i) Inter-species differences. Considerable differences in response to medicines often exist between animal species. An unequivocal response in one species may not necessarily be found at all in another. Drug actions in certain animals may be quite different from their actions in other animals. Morphine is an example: it has an almost purely depressant effect in dogs, rabbits, guinea pigs, rats, mice and birds, and a quite different, deliriant action in cats, and to a lesser extent in horses, donkeys, cattle, sheep and pigs.

(ii) Intra-species differences. Different strains within a particular animal species may show marked differences in sensitivity to a medicine. Some strains of rabbits are insusceptible to atropine and others are the opposite. The former have been shown to have significant amounts of atropine esterase in their bodies, which the latter lack. Such differences between strains within a species usually have a genetic basis, and it is important that the test group should be as far as possible genetically representative.

(iii) Sex differences. It is unusual for animal responses to medicines to differ to a major extent between the sexes, but minor differences are common. A notable and oft-quoted example is the greater sensitivity of the female rat to phenobarbitone.

(iv) Age. Young animals are often more sensitive than adults to medicines. (The same generally applies to humans.) Such differences relate to differences in distribution, metabolism and elimination; in many instances significant differences in absorption exist in the very young and there may in addition be slower metabolism, greater permeability of the blood-brain barrier, and retarded renal excretion. Very young animals and humans frequently have deficient enzyme-dependent glucuronidation systems. Occasionally, medicines may be more toxic to older animals than to the very young; ouabain is such an example. With advancing age, laboratory animals again often become more sensitive to the actions and toxicity of medicines.

(v) Husbandry. Factors such as crowding, composition of diet, and ambient temperature may materially influence the outcome of pharmacological studies in animals. In certain circumstances even slight alterations in diet may have a significant effect on drug toxicity. For some medicines a higher (or lower) than normal ambient temperature may alter their pharmacokinetics in the experimental animal, thus affecting toxicity.

(vi) Spontaneous animal diseases. Diseases may arise spontaneously in experimental animals (this can be a particular problem in long-term studies). Such diseases may influence the toxicity of medicines or confound the data with false positive results. In practice, spontaneous diseases rarely accentuate drug toxicity in animals. What can undoubtedly occur during long-term treatment in animals is that the development of spontaneous disease may be aggravated. This may bear an important influence on the findings and has particular relevance to animal studies of carcinogenicity.

1.4. Extrapolation of data from animals to man

The factors responsible for species differences in drug action, metabolism and toxicity in animals apply equally to the frequently observed differences between experimental animals and humans. Perfect correlation of animal data with human responses to medicines does not exist, nor can it be expected.

Differences in drug metabolism represent the greatest difficulty in extrapolating from animals to humans, and variation in duration of action is the commonest expression of difference. Genetically determined slow or rapid inactivation of medicines cannot be simulated in animal experiments. For example, phenylbutazone is slowly metabolised in man ($\pm 15\%$ daily), but it disappears rapidly (within a few hours) in animals such as mice, rabbits, dogs, guinea pigs and horses. (In general, biotransformation status is not related to animal size.) It is little wonder that the antirheumatic activity of this medicine was first discovered in man — enormous doses would have been required to demonstrate similar activity in rats. Pathways of detoxification of medicines may vary from one species to another, and the relative importance of a particular detoxification pathway may vary between

Table 1.1. Adverse manifestations of medicines in humans

Predictable from animal studies	Not normally predictable from animal studies
Adverse effects mediated by the actions of medicines on wrong organs, e.g. salicylates and gastrointestinal bleeding	Exaggerated effects from recommended dosage, e.g. individual sensitivity to oral anticoagulants; slow inactivation of isoniazid
Interference with natural immunity	Adverse effects predisposed to by pre-existing pathology, e.g. exacerbation of porphyria by barbiturates; drug-induced exacerbation of a previous peptic ulcer
	Drug-drug interactions
	Hypersensitivity reactions

species. Extrapolation is further complicated by the fact that it is not possible to relate rates and pathways of metabolism to the chemical structure of a medicine.

It has been suggested that sensitivity to toxic effects of medicines on target organs such as the liver, kidney and bone marrow differs in man compared with experimental animals. However, unequivocal data on the question of differences in organ sensitivity and response to toxic injury are not easy to come upon, and this point remains unclear.

Certain pharmacological actions of medicines appear to be unique to man, e.g. the effects of the ergot alkaloids in migraine, the action of the belladonna alkaloids in motion sickness, the stimulant effects of caffeine on the central nervous system, and the protective effects of fluoride in dental caries. Similarly, certain adverse drug effects in humans have not been noted and cannot be predicted in animals, while others are readily predictable from preclinical studies (Table 1.1).

Table 1.2. Surface area ratios of some common laboratory species and man (Paget, G.E. and Barnes, J.M. 1964; reproduced by permission of Academic Press, London and New York)

	20 g Mouse	200 g Rat	400 g Guinea pig	1.5 kg Rabbit	2.0 kg Cat	4.0 kg Monkey	12.0 kg Dog	70.0 kg Man
20 g Mouse	1.0	7.0	12.25	27.8	29.7	64.1	124.2	387.9
200 g Rat	0.14	1.0	1.74	3.9	4.2	9.2	17.8	56.0
400 g Guinea pig	0.08	0.57	1.0	2.25	2.4	5.2	10.2	31.5
1.5 kg Rabbit	0.04	0.25	0.44	1.0	1.08	2.4	4.5	14.2
2.0 kg Cat	0.03	0.23	0.41	0.92	1.0	2.2	4.1	13.0
4.0 kg Monkey	0.016	0.11	0.19	0.42	0.45	1.0	1.9	6.1
12.0 kg Dog	0.008	0.06	0.10	0.22	0.24	0.52	1.0	3.1
70.0 kg Man	0.0026	0.018	0.031	0.07	0.076	0.16	0.32	1.0

A common weakness in extrapolation of data between species and in comparison of dose-effect relationships is the correction of dose for body weight. A more acceptable method is to compare surface area from animal species to animal species and from animals to man (Table 1.2).

The difficulties in extrapolation from animal studies to man make it essential that the animal species investigated are as appropriate as possible. Metabolism of the medicine in the test animal compared with human metabolism of the same medicine is the most important single consideration, and details such as the route of administration, the experimental observations and the measurement of blood and tissue levels of the medicine must be as meticulously controlled as possible. There is still need for further detailed comparative metabolic studies of medicines.

1.5. Metabolite-mediated toxicity

The importance of considering metabolites of medicines in the pathogenesis of drug toxicity has been excellently reviewed by Maze and Pessayre (see Selective Bibliography).

The prediction of the toxic potential of a medicine requires a rational understanding of its metabolism. Metabolism is not necessarily synonymous with "detoxification": metabolites of foreign compounds may be carcinogenic, mutagenic or teratogenic, or they may cause tissue necrosis.

To define the role of metabolites of a medicine in its toxicity the following should be established:

(i) The metabolic pathway(s) of the medicine concerned, and the nature and relative concentrations of the metabolites formed;

(ii) Whether the toxicity of the medicine correlates better with blood and tissue concentrations of its metabolite(s) than with concentrations of the parent compound;

(iii) Whether the metabolite(s) bind covalently to susceptible tissues;

(iv) Whether a relationship exists between the site of metabolite formation and the localisation of toxicity;

(v) Whether toxicity is modified either by increasing or decreasing the rate of metabolite formation;

(vi) Whether administration of the metabolite alone produces the same toxicity as that observed after administration of the parent compound.

The liver is most directly concerned with the metabolism of medicines and foreign chemicals. Most toxic metabolites are formed in the liver, and many toxic effects occur there. Occasionally, a highly reactive metabolite forms in extrahepatic tissue and produces local toxicity. Local metabolism of potential carcinogens has been shown to be resonsible for the production of tumours of the skin and lung.

Metabolites that do not become closely bound to tissue components may diffuse from their site of formation and equilibrate with a number of other organs. Their toxicity is exerted on the tissues that are most sensitive to them. For example, methoxyflurane is defluorinated in the liver, and its toxicity, which is due to the fluoride ion, is expressed in the kidney. On the other hand, chemically reactive metabolites may be so highly unstable that they react in the same cell in which they are formed. Occasionally toxicity may be localised to the enzyme that formed the metabolite.

1.6. Early administration of medicines to man

The initial exposure of humans to a new medicine has to be carried out cautiously for several reasons. In the first place, in extrapolating preclinical animal data to man consideration has to be given to the differences that may exist between animals and humans, and man's enormous diversity of response. Certain individuals may be extremely sensitive to the pharmacological action or toxicity of a medicine. The goal of "absolute" safety can never be achieved, but can only be approached by setting a limit of acceptably low risk. After collation of all preclinical data a decision may be taken to study a new medicine in humans. The approval of regulatory authorities and an ethical review committee normally have to be obtained. Ideally the following considerations should apply to such a decision:

(a) A need for the new medicine in the treatment of a particular disease or diseases is perceived;

(b) It is considered that the new medicine may constitute a contribution to therapy;

(c) It is considered that the risks involved in the use of the new medicine for the specified indication(s) are adequately offset by its advantages.

The objectives of early administration of a new medicine to man are to establish whether it has a potentially beneficial effect; to determine details of absorption, distribution, metabolism and elimination (single-dose studies may suffice in this regard; however, single-dose studies cannot be used to predict the likely outcome of repeated dosing); to determine how the medicine acts (such information increases the reliability of pharmacological or toxicological prediction for man); and if the possibility of specific organ toxicity has been suggested by preclinical studies, further investigations, including appropriate physiological and laboratory investigations, are necessary to provide maximum information and safeguard for humans.

Pharmacologically vulnerable individuals, such as children, pregnant women, women of child-bearing age, extremely ill patients, and persons who may be subjected to particular pressure to participate in a clinical investigation or may not have proper insight into the nature of the studies, such as psychotic and mentally retarded patients and prisoners or employees, are normally excluded from early trials of new medicines.

The initial doses administered to humans are estimated from the ED_{50} of the most sensitive animal species previously investigated. The earliest dose-finding studies steadily progress from a small fraction of the predicted effective human dose. The duration of the initial dose-finding studies should not exceed the period justified as being safe by animal toxicity studies. The dose is gradually and progressively increased until an effective level is reached, or the maximum dose previously agreed upon is reached, or early unacceptable adverse effects develop, such as sedation, nausea and hypotension.

Monitoring of early administration of a new medicine to

human volunteers always includes regular clinical and laboratory evaluation including neurological examination, blood pressure monitoring, electrocardiography, and laboratory investigation of the blood count and of renal and hepatic function. For medicines scheduled for prolonged administration, trials of appropriate duration are required.

1.7. Summary and conclusions

(i) Preclinical evaluation of medicines in animals generally provides an indication of the likelihood of efficacy of a new chemical entity and a profile of its toxicity. At the same time considerable limitations exist in extrapolating animal data of efficacy and safety to humans.

(ii) Pharmacokinetic evaluation of a new medicine is important in predicting its likely safety or toxicity, including the possible toxicity of metabolites if they are pharmacologically active.

(iii) The conditions under which a new medicine is first administered to man, and the manner in which an early profile of efficacy and safety can be obtained from early studies in humans have been considered.

Selective Bibliography

Armitage P, Allen I (1950) Methods of estimating the LD_{50} in quantal responce data. J Hyg 48:298

Davey DG (1965) The study of the toxicity of potential drugs-basic principles. Proc Eur Soc Drug Toxicity (Suppl) 6:1-13

Koppanyi T, Avery MA (1966) Species differences and the clinical trial of new drugs. A review. Clin Pharmacol Ther 7:250

Lasagna L (1965) Drug toxicity in man: The problem and the challenge. Ann NY Acad Sci 123:312

Laurence DR (1965) General problems of the first administration of a potential drug to man. In: Zaimis E (ed) Evaluation of drugs in man. Pergamon Press, London

Litchfield JT (1961) Forecasting drug effects in man from studies in laboratory animals. JAMA 177:104

Maze P, Pessayre D (1976) Significance of metabolite-mediated toxicities in the safety evaluation of drugs and chemicals. In: Mehlman MA, Shapiro RE, Blumenthal H (eds) New concepts in safety evaluation, vol 1. Wiley, New York, p 307

Morrison JK, Quinton RM, Reinert H (1968) The purpose and value of LD_{50} determinations. In: Boyland E, Goulding R (eds) Modern trends in toxicology. Butterworths, London

Paget GE, Barnes JM (1964) Toxicity tests. In: Laurence DR, Bacharach AL (eds) Evaluation of drug activities: Pharmacometrics, vol 1. Academic Press, London New York

World Health Organisation (1966) Principles for preclinical testing of drug safety. WHO Tech Rep Ser 341

World Health Organisation (1975) Guidelines for evaluation of drugs for use in man. WHO Tech Rep Ser 563

Zbinden G (1963) Experimental and clinical aspects of drug toxicity. In: Garratini S, Shore PA (eds) Advances in pharmacology, vol 2. Academic Press, London New York, p 1

Zbinden G (1964) The problem of the toxicological examination of drugs in animals and their safety in man. Clin Pharmacol Ther 5:537

2 Prediction of teratogenic potential of a new medicine

2.1. Drug utilisation during pregnancy

The majority of women take medicines at some time during their pregnancy, and not infrequently pregnant women receive numerous medicines concurrently. Many of these medicines appear to be self-prescribed, and not taken on the advice of a physician. In one study the medicines most frequently taken were vitamins, acetylsalicylic acid (aspirin) and antacids, as well as over-the-counter (OTC) preparations. The OTC preparations most commonly implicated are minerals, vitamins, analgesics, antacids, iron preparations, laxatives, nasal decongestants, antihistamines, antitussives, antiemetics and sedatives.

The true extent of fetal exposure to medicines is difficult to assess. Patients often do not equate OTCs purchased without prescription with pharmacological agents, even though they are taken as treatment for a complaint.

All things considered, the incidence of teratological injury from medicines appears to be very low. This does not rule out the importance of such injury when it does occur.

It is essential that care should be taken that the fetus is not exposed to potentially harmful agents. This is the responsibility of physicians, pharmacologists and drug regulatory authorities. Pregnant women should be educated that OTC medicines may have an adverse effect on their well-being and on the well-being of their fetuses.

2.2. The thalidomide model of drug-induced fetal damage

Concepts regarding adverse effects of medicines on the developing embryo may be attributed to a considerable degree to what might be referred to as the "thalidomide model". Not only has thalidomide influenced thinking on drug safety enormously; it has also contributed to an understanding of the pathogenic mechanisms of teratogenicity. At the same time, the model has its limitations.

The thalidomide model suggests that damage to the fetus is caused at the level of susceptible fetal tissues by the toxic agent's having gained direct access to the tissues concerned. Damage is time-related, taking place at the critical period of organogenesis, which in the human embryo is approximately between the 3rd and 12th weeks of pregnancy. Taken outside this critical period thalidomide was generally regarded as harmless, although this was not necessarily the case. The organ most actively growing at the time of exposure of the embryo to the teratogen was most vulnerable. Not all fetal organs were equally susceptible to damage by thalidomide, suggesting a certain organ specificity of the teratogen. The toxic effects on the embryo were not necessarily dose-related. Severe damage was noted in the infants of women who had allegedly taken very small doses. The clinical expression of toxicity of the teratogen ranged across a continuum of mild, moderate, severe and lethal manifestations. It was considered that only a minority (an estimated 20%) of women taking thalidomide during the vulnerable period of pregnancy gave birth to deformed infants, although consensus on this point was not reached.

The principles of drug-induced teratogenesis as reflected by thalidomide are not universally applicable. Fetal damage might not necessarily be due to direct drug action on fetal organs. The major site of action of the teratogen may be a metabolic effect in the mother, with only secondary effects on the fetus, or a primary action on the placenta. It is possible that drug effects on the paternal sperm may have an adverse effect on subsequent offspring. Furthermore, drug damage is not necessarily limited to the critical period of organogenesis, although at other periods of fetal development such an association may be less easy to identify. For example, several antineoplastic drugs given in the third trimester of pregnancy may result in growth retardation of the fetus, and methyl mercury given at any stage in pregnancy may result in permanent abnormal behavioural effects. Intrauterine fetal exposure to a teratogen may produce an effect later in life. The best known example of this is vaginal adenosis and vaginal carcinoma developing in teenagers who had been exposed in intrauterine existence to diethyl stilboestrol. Many drug effects on the fetus are certainly not all-or-nothing affairs, or easily predictable. The mechanisms of drug damage that may be applicable to thalidomide may not have relevance for other teratogens.

Thorough preclinical testing of thalidomide in experimental animals for teratogenic potential — not that this was done in the case of thalidomide prior to its use in humans — would have shown that not all animal species would have developed fetal abnormalities. (Thalidomide is teratogenic in man and to a lesser degree in rabbits, whereas rat and mice embryos are not harmed by large doses.) Animal prediction is therefore limited by species specificity of response to teratogens.

2.3. The spectrum of teratogenic effects

A complete spectrum of possible degrees of damage may ensure from administering a teratogen to the pregnant human mother or to the pregnant experimental animal. Numerous factors may modify the expression and extent of the damage, as will be indicated later.

The various expressions of effect are as follows:

(i) No apparent damage. The fact that an established teratogen, given to a pregnant female at a time during her pregnancy when the fetus can be expected to be vulnerable, might not necessarily cause damage, cautions against a "single-event" approach. In predicting the effect of a teratogen its pharmacological action has to be considered in association with possible genetic and environmental modifying factors. A teratogen such as a medicine may simply act in a complementary fashion, together with other conditions, in causing fetal injury.

(ii) Structural malformations. Malformations do not occur when a teratogenic agent is administered prior to embryonic organ differentiation. Prior to organ differentiation all cells are structurally and chemically alike, and would be expected to react in a similar fashion to a toxin. If the agent is potent enough to kill or severely damage the cells, they all tend to be affected in like manner and the embryo will die. Specific structural organ defects only occur when different groups of cells have differing susceptibilities and growth potentialities.

(iii) Growth retardation, long-term psychomotor effects, and long-term behavioural effects. When teratogens are administered after the critical period of organogenesis these less obvious abnormalities of fetal development may be noted, although teratogens such as methyl mercury may cause these effects when given at any stage during pregnancy.

(iv) Fetal death. An agent capable of causing fetal malformations also invariably causes an increase in embryonic mortality. It is likely that death and abnormal development are simply different degrees of reaction to the same noxious stimulus. Whether mortality or malformation results seems to be roughly related to the dose of the toxin. Unlike the thalidomide situation, for many teratogens the evidence suggests that embryos are able to tolerate small doses without any permanent change, thus exhibiting a "margin of tolerance". Each embryo has a threshold above which irreparable changes occur. This is the teratogenic zone, which is quite narrow. A slight further increment in dose can be expected to result in fetal death. Just as the threshold for malformations rise with advancing fetal age, so also does the threshold for mortality.

The expression of a teratogenic effect depends on a variety of factors, and not all fetuses are affected in the same manner. These factors include drug dosage, duration of dosage, the stage during pregnancy of drug administration, route of drug administration to the mother, maternal and fetal genotype, and possible multiple drug exposure. These principles are as true for the experimental animal as they are for the human female.

2.4. Prediction of the teratogenic potential of a new medicine

In the evaluation of a possible teratogenic effect of a new medicine the following considerations are important:

2.4.1. Record of safety in pregnant women

The most valuable criterion of safety of a medicine with respect to teratogenicity potential is its "track record" of safety in pregnant human females, provided such data are available and have been carefully evaluated. For example, animal experimental data suggesting an association of malignant tumours of the female breast with the oral contraceptives have been effectively negated by negative epidemiological findings over the past 10-15 years.

2.4.2. Animal teratological tests

Studies of fetotoxicity in experimental animals should be regarded as essential for all new medicines. Several points are important in the execution and interpretation of such animal studies:

(i) No animal species has identical susceptibility to man with respect to teratogens. The choice of animal is, therefore, to some extent arbitrary. At least two species, one a rodent and the other not, should be studied. Ideally three different animal species are studied.

(ii) Fetal damage may be critically dependent upon drug dosage and route of administration. The selection of the doses studied is carefully considered in accordance with the pharmacological and toxicological profiles of the medicine, and a dose range is examined for its effect upon the fetus. Low or intermediate doses of a potentially fetopathogenic medicine need not necessarily produce a teratogenic effect; very high doses may be lethal to the fetus or to the mother. Thus, too low or excessively high doses may fail to reveal the true pathogenic potential of a medicine. Similarly, it cannot be said that agents which are teratogenic in high doses in animals will necessarily produce teratogenic effects in man at therapeutic dose levels. Different routes of administration may produce differences in bioavailability and metabolism; therefore, the method of administration of the medicine to experimental animals should be the same as that designed for administration to man. If different routes of administration are intended for clinical practice, teratological tests in animals should be carried out using each route.

(iii) Administration of a medicine continuously throughout pregnancy may significantly alter the mother's metabolism of the medicine and in this way possibly mask a teratogenic effect. It is preferable that doses are given to test animals at specific times during pregnancy, as well as continuously.

(iv) The range of possible effects on the animal fetus reflects a similar range of abnormalities produced by teratogens in the human fetus. This range extends from an absence of apparent adverse effect to structural malformations of organs and limbs, growth retardation, long-term psychomotor effects, long-term behavioural effects, and fetal death. Different malformations may be caused at different stages of pregnancy by the same agent.

(v) It is important that careful note is taken of infrequent fetal abnormalities in the test animals.

(vi) Careful examination of control animals is important. The controls serve to define the rate of spontaneous malformation in the animal population studied. It is essential that controls do not reveal a high incidence of abnormalities (normally a spontaneous rate of abnormalities exceeding 8-10% is regarded as being unacceptably high). There is a risk that, in such a situation, the teratogenic potential of a medicine may not be detected.

(vii) There is no absolute assurance that negative results obtained in animals necessarily exclude the possibility that an agent will have a teratogenic effect in man.

2.4.3. Structural relationship to known teratogens

New medicines with chemical profiles closely similar to known teratogenic agents should be considered with particular caution. This refers to the following two categories of human teratogens: (a) those agents for which a definite association with fetal abnormalities in humans has been demonstrated; this includes thalidomide, organic mercury, folate antagonists, androgenic hormones, anticonvulsants, antineoplastic agents, and warfarin sodium; and (b) agents for which a definite association with teratogenesis has not been proven, but the likelihood of there being such an association is considerable, e.g. antihistamines, tranquillisers, tricyclic antidepressants, and salicylates (Table 2.1).

Table 2.1. Classification of medicines according to teratogenic risk. (Source: Wilson 1979)

Known human teratogens	Suspected human teratogens	Possible human teratogens	Not believed to be teratogenic under normal conditions of use
Androgenic hormones	Alcohol (maternal alcoholism)	Anaesthetics	Barbiturates
		Antibiotics	LSD
Antineoplastic agents	Alkylating agents	Antihistamines	Marihuana
Folic acid antagonists	Anticonvulsants	Antituberculous agents	Narcotic analgesics
Organic mercury	Neurotropic-anorectic medicines	Female sex hormones	Sulphonamides
Thalidomide	Oral hypoglycaemic agents	Lithium carbonate	
	Warfarin	Quinine and other antimalarials	
		Salicylates	
		Tranquillisers	
		Tricyclic antidepressants	

2.4.4. Pharmacokinetic and pharmacodynamic characteristics

Consideration of the physicochemical characteristics of a medicine should give an indication as to whether it is likely to cross the placenta and gain access to the fetal circulation and fetal tissues in concentrations which may cause damage. Placental transfer and concentration in fetal tissues will be greatest for medicines which have a high lipid solubility, a molecular weight less than 1000, and a low proportion ionised at pH 7.4. Placental transfer will be proportional to the concentration of the unbound component for those medicines that bind significantly to plasma proteins.

Medicines which accumulate in the body, or which are administered long-term, are sometimes associated with an increased likelihood of teratogenesis. For this reason special attention is generally given to medicines which are designed for long-term or repeated intermittent use in the treatment of chronic illnesses.

Medicines which do not appear to be primarily teratogenic in their own right, or capable of crossing the placenta and gaining access to vulnerable fetal tissues, may nevertheless metabolise to potentially toxic derivatives. The main metabolic pathways and the metabolites of a medicine under scrutiny are of relevance in this regard.

Pharmacological effects on placental blood flow, endocrinological effects on the normal hormonal balance of the fetus, or tranquillising or psychotropic effects in the mother (which might be expected to affect the central nervous system of the fetus in addition) are regarded as potentially teratogenic. (Tranquillising and psychotropic agents are amongst the most likely medicines to be prescribed for women during pregnancy.)

2.5. Decision-taking in practice

It has to be accepted that in many instances precise evaluation of risk of teratogenicity of a new medicine cannot be made in preclinical and early studies in man.

There remain certain inherent difficulties in establishing that a particular medicine has teratogenic potential. These have been summarised by Smithells (see Selective Bibliography):

(i) The more widely used the medicine and the more common the malformation, the more often will they be associated by chance and the more difficult it is to establish a causal relationship;

(ii) A factor that predisposes to malformation is less easy to identify than one that causes malformation;

(iii) Methods of reporting may give a false impression of association (cases with positive histories are more likely to be reported than those with negative histories; the parents of malformed infants tend to give more frequent positive histories than the parents of healthy controls);

(iv) Controlled studies in human beings may not be carried out for ethical reasons.

In practice, women should be exposed as little as possible to medicines when they are pregnant, and careful consideration should be given to any medicines that are prescribed. On the other hand, under certain conditions the advantages of drug therapy during pregnancy may clearly outweigh the disadvantages. For example, there is evidence that antiepileptic drug therapy may be associated with an increased incidence of cleft lip and/or cleft palate and numerous other congenital malformations in the infants of epileptic women who take these medicines during their pregnancy. Animal studies with phenytoin sodium confirm a high incidence of numerous fetal skeletal and organ disorders. However, almost all physicians would agree that the effects of uncontrolled seizures may be worse than the risk of the medicines, and they stress that epileptics who require therapy should continue with it during their pregnancy.

2.6. Summary and conclusions

(i) The incidence of teratological injury caused by medicines is low. However, when this does occur the consequences may be serious. The risks of such an event should be reduced to an absolute minimum.

Conclusions

(ii) Thalidomide has contributed significantly to our understanding of drug-induced teratogenesis, but the pathogenic model which it provided is not universally applicable to other teratogens.

(iii) The spectrum of adverse effects of drugs upon the developing fetus may range from the mildest form of expression which may be subclinical to a lethal outcome, and the nature and severity of the effect is largely determined by factors relating to the administration of the drug, and maternal and fetal genotype. These principles are as true for experimental animals as they are for humans.

(iv) In the prediction of teratogenicity potential of a medicine the most valuable criterion of safety is its record in pregnant human females, provided such data are available and have been carefully evaluated.

(v) In the preclinical assessment of teratogenic potential the most important considerations are experimental animal studies and prediction of the likelihood of the medicine or its metabolite(s) gaining access in toxic amounts to fetal tissues, and for prolonged duration.

(vi) Animal studies of drug-induced teratogenicity are valuable, but extrapolation to humans is limited by important differences in the conditions pertaining to the pregnant human female. Animal investigations should simulate as closely as possible the likely situation in humans with respect to dosage, mode of administration, and pharmacokinetics.

(vii) Close structural similarity of a new medicine to a known teratogen is important, although precise prediction of teratogenic potential from physicochemical characteristics is not possible.

(viii) The decision to prescribe any medicine for a pregnant woman has to be made on the basis of risk-benefit assessment.

Selective Bibliography

Heinonen OP, Sloane D, Shapiro S (1977) Birth defects and drugs in pregnancy. Publishing Sciences Group, Littleton, Massachusetts
Smithells RW (1976) Environmental teratogens of man. Br Med Bull 32:27
Wilson JG (1959) Environmental studies on congenital malformations. J Chronic Dis 10:111
Wilson JG (1979) Embryotoxicity of drugs in man. In: Wilson JG, Clarke Fraser F (eds) Handbook of teratology, 1: General principles and etiology. Plenum Press, New York
World Health Organisation (1967) Principles for the testing of drugs for teratogenicity. WHO Tech Rep Ser 364

3 Prediction of dependence-producing potential of a new drug

3.1. The features of drug dependence in man

The clinical state of drug dependence in man is a condition of periodic or chronic intoxication produced by the repeated consumption of a drug. The characteristics of this condition include the following:

(i) An overpowering desire or need (compulsion) to continue taking the drug, and to obtain it by any means. This compulsion to take the drug on a continuous or periodic basis is in order to experience its psychic effects, and to avoid the discomfort of its absence;

(ii) A tendency to increase the dose (tolerance), which is an adaptive state in which there is a diminished response to the dose of the drug originally required to produce a particular effect. However, drug dependence may occur without the development of tolerance;

(iii) Psychic (psychological) and often physical dependence on the effects of a drug. Psychic dependence is a drive which requires periodic or chronic administration of the drug for pleasure, or to avoid discomfort. It is the most dominant feature of chronic intoxication with psychotropic drugs. In some cases psychic drive may be the only feature of drug dependence. Craving may be intense. Physical dependence is an adaptive state in which intense physical disturbances occur when administration of the drug is suspended, or when its action is counteracted by a specific antagonist. All drugs capable of producing dependence cause psychic dependence. Physical dependence may or may not be a prominent feature of drug dependence;

(iv) A detrimental effect on the individual and on society.

An individual may concomitantly be dependent on more than one drug.

3.2. Clinical profiles of drug dependence

The disturbances caused when the administration is suspended of a drug upon which a patient is dependent, or when its action is counteracted by a specific antagonist, display a spectrum of symptoms and signs which are known collectively as the abstinence or withdrawal syndrome. The withdrawal syndrome is relieved by readministration of the drug concerned or by another drug of similar pharmacological action of the same generic type, but not completely by drugs of different generic types.

Individuals may become dependent upon a wide variety of chemical substances, covering the whole range of effects on the central nervous system from stimulation to depression. The features of drug dependence show marked variations from one drug type to another, and in broad terms a pattern can be defined for each type. These patterns are sufficiently consistent to permit identification of the following types of dependence (only drugs in common medical practice are included in this list): morphine type; barbiturate type; amphetamine type; and benzodiazepine type. Dependence on drugs belonging to each of these generic groups may develop with doses of the drug within the range normally used for therapeutic purposes. The clinical profile of drug dependence is likely to be similar for closely related congeners, and the withdrawal syndrome rapidly abated by the administration of a drug belonging to the group concerned. Although a certain degree of overlap exists between groups, the clinical profiles are sufficiently characteristic for them to be regarded as separate entities.

3.2.1. Morphine-type dependence

Morphine dependence is characterised by all three distinct features of drug dependence — tolerance, habituation and physical dependence. Morphine dependence may be set in motion by the first dose administered, and it is invariably present after 2 to 3 weeks of continuous therapy. For certain congeners of morphine, such as codeine, the interval is definitely longer. This is particularly so for orally administered drugs, as opposed to those given parenterally. Both psychic and physical dependence develop early and are powerful, and they increase in intensity in parallel with an increase in dosage. Continued administration of morphine, or a congener of morphine, is required to maintain homeostasis. Variations exist in the capacity of potent morphine-like substances to induce dependence and to substitute for one another. Administration of a morphine antagonist to such patients precipitates the characteristic abstinence syndrome (Fig. 3.1).

The abstinence syndrome first manifests within several hours (approximately 6) of the last dose and reaches a peak in intensity in 24 to 48 hours. It is a self-limited condition which subsides spontaneously. The most severe symptoms usually disappear within 10 days of drug withdrawal although residual symptoms persist for a much longer period (up to 5-6 weeks). The time of onset, maximum intensity, and duration of signs and symptoms vary with the specific drug involved. The administration of a morphine antagonist to morphine-dependent patients promptly precipitates a rapid and intense syndrome that lasts only a few hours.

The morphine abstinence syndrome represents changes in all major areas of nervous activity, including alteration in behaviour, simultaneous excitation of both the sympathetic and parasympathetic divisions of the autonomic nervous system, and dysfunction of the somatic nervous system. Symptoms and signs include anxiety, restlessness, body aches, insomnia, yawning, lacrimation, rhinorrhoea, mydriasis, piloerection (gooseflesh), hot flushes, nausea, vomiting, diarrhoea, dehydration, anorexia, loss of body weight, and elevation of body temperature, respiratory rate and systolic blood pressure.

3.2.2. Barbiturate- and alcohol-type dependence

The features of chronic intoxication with barbiturates and alcohol are similar, and so are the manifestations of abstinence from these agents. Barbiturates suppress alcohol abstinence effects, and alcohol will suppress, at least partially, the symptoms of barbiturate withdrawal. These similarities justify the concept of "dependence of barbiturate-alcohol type", although there are psychological and sociological differences between the two (Fig. 3.2).

Dependence on barbiturates presents certain similarities to morphine dependence, although the pictures of intoxication and withdrawal are different. Barbiturate-dependence usually develops as a result of repeated administration of doses that generally exceed the usual therapeutic levels. Patients have a strong desire to continue taking the drug. This need can be satisfied by any drug having barbiturate-like properties. Barbiturates produce both psychic and physical dependence. Tolerance develops and may become evident within several days of initiation of treatment. In contradistinction to the situation with morphine-like drugs, there is a limit to the dose of barbiturates to which a person can become tolerant. This limit differs in individual patients and varies widely. Following withdrawal of barbiturates tolerance is rapidly lost, and some patients may subsequently be more sensitive to the drug than they may have been at the onset of treatment.

The clinical manifestations that characterise chronic barbi-

General structure:

Generic name:	R_1	R_2	R_3	Other changes[a]
Morphine	OH	–H, –OH	CH_3	—
Codeine	OCH_3	–H, –OH	CH_3	—
Heroin	$OCOCH_3$	–H, –$OCOCH_3$	CH_3	—
Hydrocodone	OCH_3	=O	CH_3	1
Hydromorphone	OH	=O	CH_3	1
Levorphanol	OH	–H, –H	CH_3	1,3
Oxycodone	OCH_3	=O	CH_3	1,2
Oxymorphone	OH	=O	CH_3	1,2
Nalorphine[b]	OH	–H, –OH	$CH_2CH=CH_2$	—
Naloxone[b]	OH	=O	$CH_2CH=CH_2$	1
Naltrexone[b]	OH	=O	$CH_2CHCH_2\underset{CH_2}{\diagdown\diagup}$	1

[a] other changes to the general structure in the morphine molecule are as follows:
1. Single instead of double bond between C_7 and C_8
2. OH added to C_{14}
3. No oxygen between C_4 and C_5

[b] antagonists

Fig. 3.1. Narcotic agonists and antagonists chemically related to morphine

turate intoxication are sedation, ataxia, impairment of mental acuity, confusion, and emotional lability. The barbiturate abstinence syndrome is distinctive. It appears within 24 hours of cessation of treatment, reaches peak intensity in 2-3 days, and subsides slowly over a matter of weeks. There is no antagonist which is known to precipitate the barbiturate abstinence syndrome while a patient is taking barbiturates. The approximate order in which the features of the abstinence syndrome appear is: anxiety, involuntary twitching of muscles, tremor, progressive weakness, dizziness, distortion of visual perception, nausea, vomiting, insomnia, weight loss, precipitous fall in blood pressure on standing, convulsions of grand-mal type, delirium resembling delirium tremens, or a major psychotic episode resembling schizophrenia with delusions and hallucinations. A withdrawn semi-stuporous state and disorganised panic have been seen. Convulsions and delirium do not usually occur before 48-72 hours after withdrawal.

There is no evidence that physical dependence of the barbiturate type is set in motion by the first dose. There is also no evidence that physical dependence develops to a significant degree with long-term continuation of therapeutic doses usual for the production of sedation or hypnosis. The dose has to be increased appreciably before signs of abstinence will appear on abrupt withdrawal. A degree of psychic dependence may develop with therapeutic doses of barbiturates, but treatment with such doses can usually be discontinued without serious disturbance.

3.2.3. Amphetamine-type dependence

The amphetamines elevate mood and induce a state of wellbeing. This is true, too, for drugs that derivatise into metabolites with amphetamine-like action. This is the reason for their widespread use as stimulants, and may partly explain their action as anorexiants. Administration is often prolonged and continuous, and varying degrees of psychic dependence may develop. Often the dose is increased in order to attain stimulation and a state of elation. Abuse of this class of drugs originates in, and is perpetuated by, the drive to obtain maximum euphoria.

The amphetamines are certain to induce tolerance. Although this develops slowly, a progressive increase in dose

General structure:

(i) Long duration of action (6 h or more)

	R_1	R_2	R_3
Barbitone	H	C_2H_5	C_2H_5
Phenobarbitone	H	C_2H_5	C_6H_5

(ii) Intermediate duration of action (3-6 h)

	R_1	R_2	R_3
Amylobarbitone	H	C_2H_5	$(CH_3)_2CHCH_2CH_2$
Butobarbitone	H	C_2H_5	C_4H_9

(iii) Short duration of action (less than 3 h)

	R_1	R_2	R_3
Hexobarbitone	CH_3	CH_3	C_6H_9
Pentobarbitone	H	C_2H_5	$CH_3CH_2CH_2\underset{\underset{CH_3}{\vert}}{C}H$
Secobarbitone	H	$CH_2=CHCH_2$	$CH_3CH_2CH_2\underset{\underset{CH_3}{\vert}}{C}H$

Fig. 3.2. Barbiturates used as sedatives and hypnotics. Dependence of the barbiturate-alcohol type is liable to occur with any of the barbiturates, but is most likely to occur with the shorter-acting barbiturates

may result eventually in the ingestion of quantities of amphetamine that may be several hundred-fold greater than the original therapeutic dose.

Oral administration of large amounts of amphetamines or amphetamine-like drugs may produce psychiatric effects of a psychotic nature, including hallucinations and delusions. Intravenous administration is even more likely to produce

Generic name	Structure
Amphetamine	Phenyl–CH_2CHCH_3 with NH_2
Chlorphentermine	Cl–Phenyl–$CH_2C(CH_3)_2NH_2$
Clortermine	Phenyl(ortho-Cl)–$CH_2C(CH_3)_2NH_2$
Diethylpropion	Phenyl–$C(=O)CH(CH_3)N(C_2H_5)_2$
Fenfluramine	Phenyl(meta-CF_3)–$CH_2CH(CH_3)NHC_2H_5$
Methamphetamine	Phenyl–CH_2CHCH_3 with $NHCH_3$

Fig. 3.3. Sympathomimetic agents with significant central stimulant activity

psychotic manifestations (the intravenous route is employed by habitués for the express purpose of obtaining bizarre mental effects, which may be associated with alteration in sexual functions, even to the point of orgasm). Abusers of amphetamines are prone to accidents due to both excitation and excessive fatigue which may break through and manifest at inopportune times. Intravenous administration is likely to cause serious antisocial behaviour.

Generic name	Structure
Phendimetrazine	2-phenyl-3-methyl-4-methyl morpholine (O, N-CH₃, C₆H₅, CH₃)
Phenmetrazine	2-phenyl-3-methyl morpholine (O, NH, C₆H₅, CH₃)
Phentermine	$C_6H_5\text{-}CH_2\text{-}C(CH_3)_2\text{-}NH_2$

All these agents have a stimulant action on the central nervous system and an anorectic effect in the treatment of obesity.
Continued administration frequently produces tolerance and a risk of dependence.

Fig. 3.3. (continued)

Abuse of the amphetamines does not cause obvious physical dependence, and there is no characteristic abstinence syndrome. At the same time, sudden withdrawal from large doses is not necessarily symptomless. Sudden withdrawal of a stimulant drug which may have masked chronic fatigue and a need for sleep may permit these conditions to reappear in exaggerated fashion. A state of psychic disturbance and possibly depression in the withdrawal period reinforces the

Generic name	Structure
Chlordiazepoxide	
Clorazepate	
Diazepam	
Lorazepam	

Fig. 3.4. The psychoactive benzodiazepines

compulsion to take the drug (Fig. 3.3). (This does not compare in magnitude with the physical withdrawal effects that occur with morphine, barbiturates, and alcohol. Withdrawal of drugs of the amphetamine type is seldom life-threatening, and the situation requires psychological rather than somatic therapy.)

Generic name	Structure
Medazepam	
Oxazepam	
Prazepam	
Temazepam	

All these benzodiazepines have central nervous system activity and a capacity under certain conditions of use to induce dependence.

Fig. 3.4. (continued)

3.2.4. Benzodiazepine-type dependence

Dependence upon benzodiazepines occurs rarely or not at all under normal conditions of clinical use. It is almost only after prolonged administration of larger doses than those normally recommended that it is seen.

There is negligible evidence from animal studies for

dependence-producing potential of the benzodiazepines. Only very large doses (up to 1000 times the normal pharmacological dose) have produced dependence in experimental animals. Tolerance has been noted in animal experiments. Thus, animal studies are of very little help in examining the potential for human dependence on the benzodiazepines at therapeutic dosage levels.

In human case studies of benzodiazepine-dependence the majority of authentic cases have taken alcohol or other drugs concurrently. Less than 50% took benzodiazepines alone. Most patients had taken doses of benzodiazepines which were at least twice and often four times those normally prescribed.

The clinical manifestations of benzodiazepine abstinence resemble those seen with sedatives, barbiturates, and alcohol. The duration of elimination of many of the benzodiazepines is substantially longer than the majority of sedatives. After withdrawal the signs of the abstinence syndrome usually develop between the third and sixth days. The effects tend to last for a shorter time and are less florid than those seen in the barbiturate-withdrawal state.

The mildest symptoms of benzodiazepine withdrawal are anxiety, apprehension, insomnia, dizziness and anorexia. When the drug has originally been prescribed for an anxiety state, it may be impossible to decide on clinical grounds whether such symptoms reflect abstinence or a recurrence of the underlying disorder due to premature withdrawal of therapy. Weaning dependent patients from benzodiazepines may be less difficult than when a comparable degree of dependence exists with other drugs.

The manifestations of more advanced degrees of physical dependence include muscular weakness or tremors, postural hypotension, hyperthermia, convulsions, and confusional states or psychoses. The more florid of these symptoms and signs are rare, even when excessive doses of benzodiazepines have been given for prolonged periods (Fig. 3.4).

3.3. Profile of a drug likely to produce dependence

The following are the important guidelines in the prediction of whether a new medicine is likely to have dependence-producing potential.

3.3.1. Clinical and epidemiological patterns

The most important pointer is the pattern of use and/or abuse of the medicine or of its close congener in the community. Such information is derived from systematic clinical and epidemiological observations. However, in a particular social setting or at a particular time, a dependence-producing drug need not necessarily have manifested itself as such. Evidence for drug dependence may appear in a community shortly after its introduction but may also develop much later. Negative epidemiological data need not necessarily be definitive in predicting dependence.

Today, controlled experiments in humans carried out to determine possible dependence of the morphine type are not ethically acceptable. In early human studies of new medicines with possible opiate-like activity the subjects should be carefully scrutinised for possible euphorigenic effects of single doses.

Long-term observations in man in the early investigation of drugs with possible dependence-producing potential are designed to detect the main features of the drug-dependent state. Such assessment is not only very important, but also most difficult. Moreover, negative results are not necessarily conclusive.

3.3.2. Proposed usage in clinical medicine

A drug with dependence-producing characteristics is most likely to manifest them when it is prescribed long-term for patients who are dependence-prone. Such individuals include subjects suffering from chronic pain, psychiatric disorders, insomnia associated with anxiety, and chronic psychological or physical illnesses. (The latter group is particularly prone to dependence of the barbiturate and benzodiazepine types.) The risk is compounded when chronic illness is combined with failure to respond to treatment. The risks of dependence are greatest when a drug with liability to cause dependence is prescribed in excessive dosage or repeatedly, or for excessively long periods of time.

3.3.3. Pharmacological category

The possibility of development of dependence is considered when a drug falls into one of the following pharmacological categories: narcotic analgesics; barbiturates (with the possible exception of phenobarbitone); amphetamines and drugs that metabolise to amphetamine-like substances in the body; and tranquillisers, including the benzodiazepines, under certain abnormal conditions of use.

Although close structural resemblance of a new drug to the opiate analgesics may suggest the likelihood of dependency, no clear indications exist of a consistency in the relation of chemical structure to dependence production. On the other hand, high analgesic potency of the central narcotic type and potential for dependence are inevitably associated and to date have never been separated in a drug.

Any drug fitting into one of the categories mentioned above can be regarded as being liable to abuse by some individuals under certain conditions. Problems of dependence may also arise with agents that only partially resemble the aforementioned prototypes. On the other hand, new psychotropic agents with only slight differences in structure from the prototypes may not necessarily have similar dependence characteristics.

3.3.4. Human pharmacology

Psychoactive drugs and drugs used for anorexigenic effects, sleep induction, or tranquilliser action may be liable to abuse. Following single-dose or repeated administration, the central nervous system effects may be apparent either as stimulation or as depression. The manifestations of such effects may include a euphorigenic effect, hallucinations, and disturbances in motor function, thinking, behaviour, perception or mood. Drugs which produce behavioural disorders at a dose level consistent with a self-administered regimen are of particular importance in this regard. Abuse is less likely to occur when the drug in question is locally irritating or when it produces adverse effects such as diarrhoea or other gastrointestinal disturbances.

The pharmacokinetic characteristics of a drug likely to produce dependence are most commonly a rapid onset of action and a tendency to remain in the body for a long period of time (usually for days).

When a drug displays evidence of cross-tolerance with psychotropic drugs which are known to induce tolerance in man, this may serve as valid evidence for the existence of a close pharmacological resemblance between the new drug and the drug with which cross-tolerance has been noted.

3.3.5. Animal studies

Animal models are available for the study of both the psychological and physical components of drug-dependence. In general, animal investigations offer an indication of possible dependence liability in man, but they fail to define the likelihood of risk at therapeutic dosage levels.

For animal studies to be relevant to the human situation, the pharmacokinetic and pharmacodynamic properties of the drug under review should be as similar as possible in the animal species investigated to those in man. When such comparisons cannot be made or are not well known, it is essential that more than one animal species should be studied.

The choice of animal species is important. Different laboratory animals appear to vary in their susceptibility to the different drugs. As a rule, rodents are of greater value than other laboratory animals in the prediction of addiction of

Table 3.1. Animal models of drug dependence

Drug	Mouse	Rat
Morphine	Characteristic abstinence effects can be produced by repeated administration, followed either by rapid withdrawal or by giving naloxone or nalorphine.	The rat is the preferred model for testing morphine dependence. "Dependence-resistant" rats can be identified — this trait appears to be genetically determined.
Barbiturates	Abrupt withdrawal after barbiturate intoxication lasting 14 days is followed by a fall in convulsive threshold. This correlates closely with the degree of dependence produced in man.	—
Amphetamine	—	—
Benzodiazepines	—	—

Table 3.1. (continued)

Monkey	Dog	General comments
The rhesus monkey develops physical dependence and drug-seeking with repeated administration of morphine. Severity may range from mild to very severe.	In the spinal dog, transected at T10-11, a characteristic syndrome is produced with repeated administration. Alterations in spinal reflexes are the most specific.	Main features of morphine withdrawal in laboratory animals are: weight loss irritability restlessness spasticity dehydration
—	Dogs are valuable models for barbiturate dependence. The abstinence syndrome may vary from mild to very severe. Correlation with man is good.	Features of the withdrawal syndrome in laboratory animals, in order of severity, are: weight loss tremors restlessness hyperthermia delirium convulsions
—	—	Tolerance develops rapidly in animals. After chronic administration withdrawal symptoms subside very rapidly. A specific abstinence syndrome is not described.
Enormous doses (approximately 1 000 × pharmacological dose) are required to produce dependence.	—	There is no direct evidence that animal studies of the various benzodiazepines have relevance to the human situation.

morphine-like drugs, and the dog is valuable in testing barbiturate-type dependence. The monkey is a useful model for physical dependence. There appears to be a place, too, for the study of the cat, rabbit and baboon in certain instances. It is important that the appropriate animal is studied when a profile of adverse effects is defined. The main characteristics of the various animal models of drug dependence are shown in Table 3.1.

A drug capable of suppressing a withdrawal syndrome in abstinent drug-dependent animals can be regarded as supporting physical dependence of that particular drug type.

As a rule, for physical or psychological dependence to be demonstrated in animals a drug must have two properties:

(i) It must be capable of inducing primary dependence when administered at the appropriate doses and time intervals for an appropriate period of time;

(ii) It must have the capacity to substitute for a known, related, dependence-producing agent in animals which are dependent upon that agent.

3.4. Strategy in evaluation of dependence-potential

The following steps are indicated in gathering information concerning the likelihood of dependence potential of a new drug:

(i) Structural and molecular similarities to morphine, barbiturates, amphetamines and benzodiazepines are identified. Drugs falling into one of these categories are regarded as having the potential to cause dependence.

(ii) The pharmacokinetics of a drug acting on the central nervous system are examined with special attention to a rapid onset of action combined with prolonged retention in the body.

(iii) A review is made of the pharmacological properties of the drug concerned along the lines indicated in Table 3.2.

Table 3.2. Pharmacological evaluation of dependence-producing potential

---

1) Comparison of the effects of different routes of administration
2) Potency, compared with congeners
3) Profile of adverse effects
4) Consequences of administration of a specific antagonist, if it exists
5) Determination of the rate and extent of increase of dose required during chronic administration to maintain the original pharmacological effect
6) Cross-tolerance with other drug types

(iv) An assessment is made of the degree of dependence upon the drug or its close congeners in the community. This is the most important of all criteria, when findings are available.

(v) Unless sufficient epidemiological evidence exists to the contrary, the dependence potential of any new medicine with a psychotropic action should be determined by means of appropriately planned animal investigations.

(vi) Proposed usage in "high-risk" or dependence-prone subjects should heighten caution concerning a new agent.

3.5. Summary and conclusions

(i) Drug dependence is always characterised by a compulsion to take the drug in order to experience its psychic effect; marked physical dependence and tolerance may or may not be features of the drug-dependent state.

(ii) The characteristics of drug dependence show variations from one generic drug group to another, and in practice several different profiles of drug dependence can be identified: morphine and its congeners; the barbiturates; amphetamine and its congeners; and the benzodiazepines. The abstinence syndrome is relieved partially or completely by readministration of the drug or another drug with similar pharmacological action of the same generic type, but not normally by drugs of different generic types.

(iii) A drug likely to produce dependence in man will have at least one of the following pharmacological characteristics: molecular properties similar to one of the prototypic types — morphine, barbiturates, amphetamine or benzodiazepines; a stimulant or depressant action on the central nervous system; and a prolonged duration of action or tendency to accumulate in the body, associated with a rapid onset of action.

(iv) Animal studies are useful in the evaluation of dependence-producing potential, provided the pharmacokinetics and the pharmacological action(s) of the drug in the animals which are studied resemble reasonably closely the action(s) and fate of the drug in man.

(v) In clinical practice, certain individuals may be identified as "dependence-prone" or high-risk patients. In a community the degree of dependence produced by a particular drug may vary quite significantly from one period of time to another, depending upon doctors' prescribing patterns and upon availability to and usage by the public. A health hazard exists when the problems and consequences of drug dependence extend beyond a limited number of individuals.

Selective Bibliography

Bewley TM (1972) Drug dependence caused by medical treatment. In: Meyler L, Peck HM (eds) Drug-induced diseases, vol 4. Excerpta Medica, Amsterdam, p 571

Eddy NB, Halbach H, Isbell M, Seevers MH (1965) Drug dependence: Its significance and characteristics. Bull WHO 32:721

Halbach H, Eddy NB (1963) Tests for addiction (chronic intoxication) of morphine type. Bull WHO 28:139

Marks J (1978) The benzodiazepines. Use, overuse, misuse, abuse. MTP Press, Lancaster, England

World Health Organisation (1964) Evaluation of dependence-producing drugs. WHO Tech Rep Ser 287

4 Prediction of carcinogenic potential of a new medicine

4.1. The risks of drug-induced neoplasia in man

A chemical carcinogen is a substance which induces in mammalian species tumours that are not normally encountered, or which increases the incidence of naturally occurring tumours, or which causes the appearance of naturally occurring tumour types earlier than would be expected.

It has been estimated that 80% of carcinomas in animals and humans have an exogenous cause. More than 150 chemicals have been shown to cause cancer in animals under experimental conditions, and the United States Food and Drug Administration has listed some 2400 suspected carcinogens in animals. In man there is reasonable evidence of association of only 25-30 chemicals with carcinogenesis. This means that by no means all chemicals capable of causing cancer in experimental animals are necessarily carcinogenic to man. On the other hand, with the possible exception of arsenic, all carcinogenic agents in man have been shown to produce cancer in experimental animals.

There are several reasons for the differences in susceptibility to carcinogens between experimental animals and humans. The most obvious is that in drug-induced carcinogenesis, as in other aspects of drug-induced damage, notable inter-species differences exist. Furthermore, animal experiments may be carried out in completely artificial circumstances *vis-à-vis* the situation that may apply to humans. The conditions of the animal experiments may significantly modify the expression of carcinogenic potential of a chemical. Finally, an association of chemical carcinogenicity in the human may indeed exist but not be established, because the rarity of the association may make it difficult to diagnose against "background noise" produced by limitations in history taking, clinical investigation, and epidemiological methods. A relatively short duration of observation in man may fail to reveal an association with tumour formation for a carcinogen with a very long latent period. (In certain instances 15 years may be regarded as short duration of exposure.)

Several other points are relevant to inter-species and inter-individual variations of expressions of chemical carcinogens. The effect of a carcinogen may depend upon its access to a target organ, and this may vary according to species; for example, drug passage through mouse skin is considerably greater than through human skin. For this reason the mouse is a sensitive test animal for carcinogens which pass through the skin, and this has led to misleading results. Certain carcinogens may be produced by metabolism in one organ before acting on a different target organ. Such metabolism may vary from individual to individual and from species to species, and it may depend upon the presence or absence of specific enzyme systems or on environmental factors such as diet. Certain chemical carcinogens depend for their effect on the availability of co-carcinogens which facilitate the biochemical change that converts them to active agents. Again, inter-species differences exist in the availability of co-carcinogens. The primary effect of many carcinogens is to damage DNA, which may or may not subsequently repair. Whether DNA repair takes place is genetically determined.

The association between human host and carcinogen is a dynamic one, changing with clinical and epidemiological circumstances. In the case of potentially carcinogenic medicines, variations in dose strengths, patterns of administration and combinations may vary in different therapeutic regimens, and there may be a greater risk with one regimen than with another. These considerations form the basis for the steps normally taken to evaluate carcinogenic potential prior to and following release of a medicine for use in humans.

4.2. Profile of the high-risk medicine

Several characteristics of a medicine and its clinical usage may categorise it as being high-risk with respect to carcinogenic potential in humans, particularly when there is an association of more than one of these factors.

4.2.1. Chemical structure

If a chemical is a powerful electrophilic reactant, it should be regarded as intrinsically carcinogenic. Sulphur mustard is such an example. Electrophilic reactants attach to target molecules in vulnerable cells, complexing with cellular macromolecules. The consequent damage to the cell may result in any of the following: repair, cell death, cell mutation or cellular transformation with potential carcinogenesis.

If a chemical can be shown to be metabolised in man or in animals to any degree to an electrophilic reactant, it may be regarded as potentially carcinogenic. Aflatoxin B_1 is rapidly and exclusively metabolised in a variety of species to an electrophilic reactant; nitrosamines and dialkyltriazines derivatise to electrophilic reactants along their major metabolic pathways.

A definite association exists only between a small number of medicines and cancer in humans. These include arsenic, coal tar and its derivatives, oestrogens, and immunosuppressive and antimitotic agents. New medicines which have a close structural relationship with proven carcinogens might be anticipated themselves to be potentially carcinogenic. However, in the main there has been little success in relating chemical structure to carcinogenic activity. At the same time it can be said that polycyclic aromatic hydrocarbons, aromatic amines and their derivatives, nitrosamines, alkylating agents and radiomimetics may well be carcinogenic and they should be extensively tested before use. Certain natural products also require careful attention. Apart from the aflatoxins, carcinogenic activity has been demonstrated in the metabolites of certain moulds, pyrolizidine alkaloids, and other medicines derived from plant products or susceptible to fungal contamination. Other systemically acting carcinogens include: urethan, which is carcinogenic for the lung and for a number of other organs; dimethylnitrosamine, which is carcinogenic for the liver and kidney, and certain analogues of dimethylnitrosamine which are carcinogenic to the oesophagus; and various chlorinated compounds which are toxic to and potentially carcinogenic to the liver.

The example of the ß-blockers is illustrative. Many compounds of this type have been marketed and there is no evidence that any are carcinogenic in man. However, certain ß-blockers have caused tumours in animals. As a result some regulatory authorities have insisted that no clinical work with a new ß-blocker may be instituted without prior tests having shown it to be free of a carcinogenic effect in animals (Table 4.1).

4.2.2. Pharmacokinetic characteristics

Two aspects of the pharmacokinetics of a medicine may suggest carcinogenic potential:

(i) If the medicine is retained for a long time in the body and is likely to accumulate in toxic amounts, particularly if in addition there is suspicion attaching to it concerning a close structural relationship to a known carcinogen;

(ii) If the medicine metabolises in the body to a metabolite

Human carcinogens

Table 4.1. High, medium and low risk carcinogens. (Adapted from Roe 1966)

High risk	Medium Risk	Low Risk
Alkylating agents, e.g. nitrogen mustards	Chloramphenicol	Cocarcinogenic agents including phenols, essential oils, and surface active agents
Arsenic	Griseofulvin	
Busulphan	Iron dextran	
Chlorambucil	Phenylbutazone	Cyclamates
Chlornaphazin	Tannic acid	Methotrexate
Combined corticosteroid and immuno-suppressive drug therapy		Progesterone and oral contraceptives
		Reserpine
Creosote and coal tar		
Melphalan		
Nitrosamines		
Oestrogens		
Pentamethylphos-phoramide		
Pronethalol		
ß-Propiolactone		
Tretamine		
Urethan		

or metabolites which have close structural similarities to a known carcinogen.

Many carcinogens are only active at a limited number of organs. Other carcinogens are metabolites which have been formed either at their site of action or at a distant organ, in which case the active principle is transported to its site of action. Such metabolism and transport are usually subject to individual and species variations.

4.2.3. Pharmacological action

Medicines known to affect fertility or embryogenesis, to exert hormonal effects, or to cause proliferative changes or growth in tissues should be regarded as potentially carcinogenic under certain circumstances of usage in humans.

4.2.4. Clinical and epidemiological evidence

"At-risk" clinical situations for the use of a medicine with possible carcinogenic potential are long-term or repeated intermittent administration, patient exposure to high concentrations, and proposed use in particularly "sensitive" individuals such as infants, children, pregnant women and fetuses.

When available, epidemiological data in humans represent the strongest evidence of the likelihood or otherwise of carcinogenicity of a medicine. To be meaningful such data require that human exposure has been under relevant circumstances, with the appropriate dosage of the medicine concerned. Occasional case reports may be of value in providing a lead. The use of epidemiological data in the formation of predictions is considered in Chapter 6.

4.3. Animal studies

New medicines which on grounds of the above considerations can be regarded as being extremely unlikely to have a carcinogenic action in man probably need not be submitted to exhaustive animal testing before their controlled release to man. Any medicine which has characteristics suggesting a possible risk of carcinogenicity should be fully investigated in experimental animals before it is given to humans.

Despite the fact that many millions of small animals and thousands of larger ones have been studied in attempts to detect carcinogenic activity of medicines prior to their use in man, exhaustive preclinical studies in animals of carcinogenesis are not warranted in every case of a new medicine. Such an approach can be prohibitively expensive and is ethically unacceptable, in terms of wastage of animals. Animal studies for carcinogenicity can reasonably be restricted to medicines or to clinical situations where a risk is considered to exist.

Nearly all human carcinogens are also carcinogenic in laboratory animals provided the animal tests are conducted properly. The converse is often not the case, although the possibility does exist that rarely man may be more sensitive than laboratory animals to carcinogenic agents. In an experimental animal treated with a chemical agent in which a tumour appears, this can be thought of in terms of a function of the intrinsic characteristic of the test compound, the dose administered, the duration of exposure, and the induced impairment of the animal's normal defence against cancer.

Strictly speaking, true carcinogens may be differentiated from co-carcinogens or carcinogens of the initiating or promoting type which can be regarded as having incomplete carcinogenic activity. However, there do not appear to be many substances which have been shown to take an active part in carcinogenesis as initiators or promotors and which have not subsequently been shown to be carcinogenic in their own right.

In the evaluation of carcinogenicity studies in animals detailed attention to the following is important:

(i) Control groups are required to define the expected incidence of spontaneously occurring tumour types in the animal species being tested. Certain carcinogens initiate tumour formation *de novo*; others may have the effect of increasing the incidence of spontaneously occurring tumour types, such as pulmonary tumours in mice. Any appreciable incidence of spontaneous tumours in the controls (for example, an incidence greater than 4%-5%) results in a considerable loss of the power of a test to distinguish a carcinogen from an inactive compound unless vast numbers of animals are studied. Conversely, it may be argued that if test animals have a very low spontaneous incidence of tumours it may be because they are inherently "resistant" to carcinogenesis and are unable to respond to carcinogenic chemicals. This latter biological contention is unsupported.

(ii) The ideal laboratory animal for investigation would be one in which the pharmacological action and the absorption, distribution, metabolism and elimination of the medicine being examined resemble as closely as possible the action and fate of the medicine in humans. It is not often possible to achieve this. Because of lack of close correlation, at least two animal species are normally studied; it is preferable that there should be three. Mice, rats, hamsters or dogs are normally chosen, and where possible the kinetics and the action of the compound in the test animal should compare reasonably with the situation in man. (Guinea pigs and rabbits are of limited use in carcinogenicity testing, and they are not normally employed. Monkeys are sensitive to a variety of carcinogens, but they do not offer special advantages in the majority of cases. Hamsters may be more suitable than rats or mice for testing certain aromatic amines, and the dog is recommended for testing bladder carcinogens of the aromatic amine group.) If a drug is believed to be a potential carcinogen, the test animals have to be chosen without knowledge of the manner in which the drug is metabolised in man. If administration to man becomes permissible later, it is important that its metabolism in the animals which were studied and in humans should be compared before final evaluation of carcinogenic potential is made.

(iii) Details of the experimental plan and procedure are important. Both sexes of the experimental animal should be studied. A range of doses should be evaluated, with a minimum of three dose levels. The highest dose should be 50-100 times the equivalent of the clinical dose planned for use in man, unless that dose is likely to be very toxic or fatal to the experimental animal. Very high doses may cause an established tumour to grow more rapidly or to metastasise, whereas smaller doses may initiate a malignant process. It may be possible to define a dose level for which no carcinogenic effect is produced.

Details of the number of animals required for a particular experiment have been carefully analysed by Salsburg (see Selective Bibliography). In practice, a global total of approximately 500 animals of each test species was recommended by Salsburg.

Long-term animal studies are the mainstay of carcinogenicity testing; very little information can be obtained from short-term testing. On the other hand, in rodents older than 18 months the number of controls that develop spontaneous tumours increases rapidly, and this number becomes formidable if microscopic tumours are included. In larger animals such as monkeys and dogs hormones may take up to 18 years before their carcinogenic effects may be detected.

The route of administration should be appropriate to the method of administration proposed for humans. The tissues and organs of the experimental animal should be exposed to concentrations of the medicine and its metabolites at least as high as, and preferably higher than, the levels to which human tissues are likely to be exposed. Ideally tissue concentrations of the medicine should be determined, unless other evidence makes this unnecessary.

(iv) Details of husbandry of the experimental animals are important in the evaluation of carcinogenicity data. The quantity of diet, the absence from it of naturally occurring carcinogens, the absence of crowding of animals, and the control of ambient air, water additives, pesticides and ultraviolet light are all important. These factors may influence the development of carcinoma in laboratory animals.

(v) Full necropsies are performed on all animals. Experienced pathologists are required to evaluate macroscopic and histopathological changes in order to avoid faulty interpretation of histological tumour types.

As far as is possible, differentiation is made between gross malignant tumours, benign tumours and hyperplastic lesions, as opposed to microscopic lesions. If the designation "tumour-bearing" is allowed to include microscopic lesions and tumours which are not life-threatening, the background incidence of tumours in the control animals may be so high as to reduce inappropriately the likelihood of a tumour-producing effect being noted.

4.4. Interpretation of animal data

Animal carcinogenicity testing is only sensitive enough to distinguish a fairly marked effect such as three- or four-fold increases above the background incidence of neoplasms. Increasing the number of animals in each dose group results in relatively little improvement of this statistic, unless an enormously large number of animals is used, which would be prohibitively expensive and unmanageable.

Provided reasonable care is taken to ensure that circumstances of dosage, route of administration, and drug metabolism and distribution are appropriate, reasonable extrapolation can often be made from animal studies to humans. Positive evidence is easier to obtain than negative evidence. In the latter case the animal species chosen or conditions of the experiments may have been inappropriate.

Authentic negative results may simply indicate that animals may be less sensitive than humans to the particular carcinogen. This circumstance is most unusual. Medicines and chemicals for which epidemiological evidence of carcinogenicity in humans exists are almost invariably carcinogenic to experimental animals.

The target organ of a carcinogen may vary from animal species to species, and from animals to man. Tumour formation in experimental animals in one particular organ does not necessarily mean that humans will have the same organ sensitivity to the carcinogen concerned. For example, development of the mouse lung tumour in response to a chemical carcinogen (a common mouse response) serves simply to identify the carcinogenic characteristic of the test agent and in no way reflects on the likely organ or organs at risk in humans. Ideally all animal investigative data concerning experimental carcinogenesis from all sources should be pooled and made accessible to all investigators, so that the extent of animal experimentation world-wide could be reduced to a minimum.

4.5. In vitro tests

Hundreds of new chemical entities are introduced each year for industrial, household and medicinal use. It is plainly uneconomical and not feasible to subject each of these to animal tests for carcinogenicity. Furthermore, animal tests may take up to 18 months to 2 years in rodents, and 18 years in dogs. During this period potentially useful agents may be unavailable for use.

The obvious advantages of short-term in vitro tests, using either cellular transformation or mutagenicity systems, are that animals are not subjected to investigation and the use of human material or its equivalent may obviate problems of species specificity. Such methods are much less expensive than animal experimentation, and conceivably medicines could be released earlier for clinical use.

For these reasons cellular transformation and mutagenicity studies have been undertaken extensively in recent years. However, they have never resulted in the detection of a previously unsuspected carcinogen. Their main drawbacks are that certain chemicals are converted metabolically in vivo to metabolites with carcinogenic activity. Such metabolism may not take place in cultures or during in vitro mutagenicity testing, giving rise to false-negative results. Conversely, carcinogens that are rapidly inactivated in vivo may produce false-positive results in cell culture.

Uncertainties exist therefore in interpreting positive findings in vitro and there is a risk that negative findings may be uncritically accepted as evidence of non-carcinogenicity.

4.6. Summary and conclusions

(i) Medicines most likely to induce carcinoma in humans are likely to have one or more of the following characteristics: highly reactive electrophilic properties, making the medicine or its metabolite(s) likely to attach to cellular macromolecules, with consequent damage to the cell; close structural resemblance of the medicine or its metabolite(s) to known human carcinogens; a tendency for the medicine or its metabolite(s) to accumulate in toxic amounts in the body or to persist for long periods in the body; a pharmacological action which includes an effect on fertility or embryogenesis, or a hormonal effect, or stimulation of proliferative changes or growth in tissues.

(ii) In the evaluation of potential carcinogenesis, animal studies are meaningful only when the absorption, distribution, metabolism and elimination of the medicine being investigated compare reasonably in the experimental animal and in man. Control animals should have a low incidence of spontaneously developing tumours, failing which there is a considerable loss of power of a test to differentiate a carcinogen from an inactive compound.

(iii) In vitro tests for carcinogenicity are limited in value by the large number of false-positive and false-negative reactions which is seen with these tests.

Selective Bibliography

Berenblum I (ed) (1969) Carcinogenicity testing. International Union Against Cancer; U.I.C.C. Technical Report Series, 2

Clayson DB (1962) Chemical carcinogenesis. Churchill, London

National Cancer Institute (1976) Guidelines for carcinogen bioassay in small rodents. Technical Report Series, 1. U.S. Department of Health, Education and Welfare, National Institutes of Health

Roe FJC (1966) The relevance of preclinical assessment of carcinogenesis. Clin Pharmacol Ther 7:77

Salsburg D (1978) Lifetime carcinogenic studies in rodents, viewed from the standpoint of experimental design: Weaknesses and alternatives. In: Dayan AD, Brimblecombe RW (eds) Carcinogenicity testing: Principles and problems. MTP Press, Lancaster, England, p 89

Schmahl D, Thomas C, Auer R (1977) Iatrogenic carcinogenesis. Springer, Berlin Heidelberg New York

World Health Organisation (1969) Principles for the testing and evaluation of drugs for carcinogenicity. WHO Tech Rep Ser 426

World Health Organisation (1971) Evaluation and testing of drugs for mutagenicity: Principles and problems. WHO Tech Rep Ser 482

5 The prediction of adverse drug interactions

5.1. The incidence and spectrum of drug-drug interactions

A drug-drug interaction is a pharmacological effect observed when two or more medicines are administered simultaneously and which cannot be explained by the combined action of the medicines concerned. Not all drug-drug interactions are necessarily adverse, and there may be several possible sequelae of such interactions:

(i) No significant clinical effect, or a very low incidence and magnitude of clinical effects of any kind. In this case the risk of potential harm in practice is very slight indeed. Many drug-drug interactions fall into this category.

(ii) The interaction may be beneficial, and desired by the physician; for example, the synergistic effect of two antibiotics in the treatment of severe infections.

(iii) Diminution in efficacy. This may be an important result of a drug-drug interaction, and can have more serious consequences than an alteration in toxicity. For example, there is evidence that the reliability of the oral contraceptive pill may be diminished if other medicines, such as antiepileptic agents, are used concomitantly. Several other examples exist of one medicine increasing the metabolism of another by stimulation of the activity of hepatic enzymes, and in this manner reducing the efficacy of the second.

(iv) An adverse interaction, which has an effect which is detrimental to the patient. For categorisation as an adverse drug-drug interaction such an effect should have been well documented. Its incidence may range from common to rare. The results may be mild, moderate or severe in intensity.

Much has been written of the hazards of using two or more medicines together, either as separate entities or in the form of a combination. The importance of drug-drug interactions has often been overestimated, and fortunately adverse interactions are unusual. When they do occur, most patients suffer only mild effects. However, a small number of drug-drug interactions may have serious consequences, which may occasionally be fatal. For this reason drug interactions deserve careful consideration. In predicting the safety of a medicine its possible interaction with other medicines which may be given inadvertently or intentionally with it should be anticipated as far as is possible. Differentiation has to be made between "potential" and "clinically significant" interactions. Estimates of adverse effects due to drug interactions detected by intensive hospital monitoring systems vary from 6·9% to 22%.

Adverse drug interactions can further be qualified as being of two distinct types: those in which two or more medicines with similar pharmacological actions have a cumulative effect which may be toxic, and those in which the interaction is indirect, i.e. there is an alteration in the pharmacological effect of one or both of the medicines concerned.

5.2. Clinically important adverse drug interactions

Of the clinically important adverse drug interactions, probably more than 90% are due to cumulative effects on vulnerable organ systems.

The adverse cumulative effects which are most common in practice are:

(i) Central nervous system depression due to the simultaneous administration of medicines with a depressant effect on the central nervous system, e.g. a narcotic analgesic given together with an antidepressant agent, or the cumulative effect of a barbiturate taken together with ethyl alcohol. The elderly are particularly susceptible to the adverse effects of combined therapy with medicines affecting the central nervous system. Sedation, confusion, disorientation, disinhibition reactions, and aggressive outbursts are common symptoms of combined drug affects in the elderly. There may be syncope and loss of consciousness. Considering the ease with which many elderly patients develop organic confusional psychoses when hypoxia, infection, or cerebrovascular incidents occur, it is not surprising that combination drug therapy causes similar adverse psychiatric effects.

(ii) Depression of the cardiovascular system by the combined effects of two medicines both acting on the heart. The reasons for such combined adverse effects are not hard to discern. Many cardiovascular medicines have a narrow therapeutic range, a steep dose-response relationship, and an action which forces itself upon the physician's attention. The most notable effects of such cumulative action are hypotension, severe bradycardia, and blockade of the cardiac conducting system. An example of such an interaction is the additive effect of ß-blocking agents and quinidine in their inhibitory effects on atrio-ventricular conduction, which may produce or aggravate already existing heart block.

(iii) Other examples are the additive anticholinergic actions of tricyclic antidepressants and phenothiazines, or antihistamines, which may lead to troublesome urinary retention, dry mouth and loss of visual accommodation. Occasionally, marked anticholinergic activity and central nervous system effects may ensue. Drug interactions of this kind may occur in an insidious manner, through ignorance of what proprietary preparations contain. Proprietary preparations may contain an antihistaminic or a phenothiazine.

Cumulative blood sugar depression, cytotoxic and bone-marrow depressant effects, and cumulative bronchoconstriction may result from the simultaneous administration of two or more medicines with similar actions.

As opposed to cumulative effects, adverse reactions due to altered pharmacokinetics of one medicine caused by another tend as a rule to be less prominent clinically. However, in certain circumstances they may be no less important. This applies particularly to the oral anticoagulants of the coumarin group, which stand out among all other medicines in this regard. There are several reasons for this. The coumarin anticoagulants are often given to patients over long periods, and patients are likely to receive other medicines concurrently. Medicines such as diuretics, hypoglycaemic agents, sedatives, hypnotics, analgesics, and acidic non-steroidal anti-inflammatory agents may interact with the oral anticoagulants. In contrast to the situation with many other medicines, the exact intensity of the pharmacological effect of a coumarin anticoagulant is important during therapeutic use. The magnitude of the pharmacological action of the oral anticoagulants is routinely and reliably monitored during their therapeutic use. Furthermore, the concentrations of the coumarins can be determined in plasma. For these reasons, drug interactions with oral anticoagulants are not only common, but they are often therapeutically important and may be serious. They are also comparatively easy to detect and analyse (Table 5.1).

5.3. Prediction of adverse drug interactions

Before a new medicine is made freely available, consideration should be given to other medicines which might be given concurrently. Ideally it should be ascertained that one does not exacerbate the toxicity of the other. It is not possible to

Table 5.1. Clinically important adverse drug-drug interactions

Interacting medicines		Effect of interaction	Clinical consequence
Coumarin anticoagulants	Phenylbutazone (and other acidic antiinflammatory agents)	Transient increase in free plasma level of coumarin	Exaggerated bleeding
Coumarin anticoagulants	Barbiturates	Induction of hepatic microsomal enzymes by barbiturates, with resultant increased metabolism of the coumarins	Exaggerated bleeding after discontinuation of barbiturate following combined therapy
Digitalis	Diuretic therapy (with associated potassium loss)	Hypokalaemia; increased sensitivity to digitalis	Digitalis toxicity
Monoamine oxidase inhibitors	Amphetamine (and other sympathomimetic agents)	Noradrenaline accumulation at receptor sites	Hypertensive crisis
Morphine (and other narcotic analgesic agents)	Tricyclic antidepressants Barbiturates (and other central nervous system depressants)	Central nervous system depression	Coma Respiratory failure
Quinidine (and other cardiac depressants)	ß-Blockers	Combined depression of cardiac conduction	Heart block
Tolbutamide	Phenylbutazone	Inhibition of tolbutamide metabolism	Severe hypoglycaemia
Tricyclic antidepressants	Sympathomimetic agents	Blocked reuptake of catecholamines at nerve terminal	Acute hypertension

Adapted from: 1. World Health Organization (1968) Principles for the clinical evaluation of drugs. Technical Report Series No.403. WHO, Geneva. 2. Hansten PD (1979) Drug interactions. Lea and Febiger, Philadelphia cater for all contingencies, but likely drug-drug effects should be anticipated.

A standard protocol for evaluation of drug interactions is not recommended as it is recognised that the investigative approach might vary according to the characteristics of the medicines involved and the projected circumstances of use. There may be more than one mechanism of adverse interaction of two specific medicines, and these mechanisms may be varied and complex. Several medicines may both potentiate and antagonise the effect of other medicines at the same time. (For example, phenobarbitone given together with tolbutamide might displace the latter from serum protein binding sites, thus releasing a disproportionately high concentration of free plasma tolbutamide, while at the same time, by induction of hepatic microsomal enzymes, the phenobarbitone may accelerate the metabolism of tolbutamide.) For these reasons, classifications of mechanisms of interaction and assessment based upon mechanisms are at risk of being an oversimplification. It is therefore undesirable to make all-embracing statements about the manner in which one medicine may affect another. Precise definition of the interaction of two medicines is always necessary.

Certain categories of medicines with common therapeutic action are particularly liable to be implicated in adverse drug interactions. These include antidepressant agents, analgesics, oral anticoagulants, oral hypoglycaemics, and sympathomimetic and antihypertensive medicines. Medicines most likely to be administered in conjunction with OTC products might be added to this category. It is these categories that should receive the most careful evaluation for potential interactions with other medicines.

The investigative approach depends upon the characteristics of the medicines concerned and the projected circumstances of use.

5.3.1. Pharmacokinetic and pharmacodynamic characteristics

Several pharmacokinetic and pharmacodynamic characteristics may serve as indicators that drug-drug interactions may be likely or that their effects may be significant. These include the following:

(i) Narrow therapeutic margin. There is a definite risk of an adverse interaction when a medicine is harmful in excess and at the same time it has a narrow therapeutic margin. Examples of such medicines include the hypoglycaemic agents, oral anticoagulants, digitalis preparations, medicines with depressant action on the central nervous system, and the cytotoxics. The addition of a further medicine may adversely modify the pharmacokinetic characteristics or the action of the medicine at receptor level, thus increasing the potential for toxicity.

(ii) Plasma protein binding. Acidic medicines which bind extensively (e.g. greater than 95% to 97%) to plasma proteins and which may be displaced by other medicines of an acidic nature, thus releasing potentially toxic amounts of free drug in the plasma, should be regarded as a "risk group" in terms of likely interactions with other medicines. The best-known examples in this category are the non-steroidal anti-inflammatory analgesic agents and the oral anticoagulants.

(iii) Toxic metabolite formation. For those medicines which metabolise to produce potentially toxic derivatives, the addition of another medicine which might induce or augment such metabolism, or alter metabolic pathways so that increased amounts of a toxic metabolite are produced may have important consequences. An example is paracetamol, which derivatises in the body to several metabolites, at least one of which is hepatotoxic. In the event of another medicine being given simultaneously which might augment this metabolic pathway (no such example has definitely been demonstrated in man) a potentially dangerous interaction might be anticipated.

Prediction of the practical significance of induction of the metabolism of one medicine by another may be complicated by the fact that the effects of the inducing agent may be either inhibitory or stimulatory in different circumstances. The magnitude and duration of alteration of the metabolism of a medicine caused by an inducer will depend upon factors such as the time interval between the administration of the medicine and the inducer. The effects of inducers with long half-lives which attain high blood levels may be particularly difficult to predict. If a medicine is normally metabolised rapidly or undergoes metabolism by several independent routes, then induction may not necessarily cause significant modifications in its toxicity profile. However, if in an individual patient the blood levels of a medicine or its metabolites are critical for therapeutic efficacy or safety, induction of metabolite formation may have important consequences.

(iv) Common toxicological profiles. When two medicines have similar pharmacological mechanisms and act at the same or similar tissue sites, their simultaneous administration may result in unwanted exaggerated effects and toxicity. Medicines with depressant action on the central nervous and cardiovascular systems are important examples.

Here it should be mentioned that extrapolation between closely related pharmacological agents may prove unwise. Minor modifications in chemical structure can result in considerable changes in pharmacokinetic and pharmacodynamic characteristics, and hence in toxicity and the possibility of interaction with other medicines. Prediction is made more difficult by the fact that medicines with closely related profiles of pharmacological action and toxicity may differ in biotransformation, molecular binding, and passage into tissues.

5.3.2. Animal studies
Animal studies are of strictly limited value in anticipating

Animal studies

adverse drug-drug interactions in man, mainly because of the difficulty in extrapolating findings from experimental animals to man, due to species differences, and the usual discrepancies in pharmacokinetics between experimental animals and humans. Great caution is therefore necessary in predicting clinical consequences of drug-drug effects from data derived from animal models, and the significance for man of most interactions noted in animals remains unclear.

There is a further reason why drug interactions observed in the laboratory animal might fail to manifest themselves at the bedside. Interactions involving medicines possessing a wide safety margin, or medicines producing therapeutic effects that are difficult to quantify accurately may often remain undetected clinically.

Having stressed their limitations, brief reference may be made to the following recognised procedures for animal testing of drug-drug interactions:

(i) LD_{50}. The determination of LD_{50} is the most commonly performed animal experiment in this regard. It is frequently required for determining the toxicological profile of fixed-ratio combination medicines, and it may also give an indication of the possibility of an adverse reaction when two medicines are given together.

The LD_{50} experiment must be carried out using the same route of administration as that prescribed for man. A rodent species is normally used. In fixed-ratio studies the single components and the combination should be tested in the same experiment. It is usually necessary to test the combination at more than one dosage level. The absorption and elimination kinetics of medicines in the rodent are generally different from those in man and pharmacological interactions may differ depending upon the relationships of blood and tissue levels; therefore ideally more than one animal species is examined in this manner.

For the selection of dose ratios the procedure of Chen and Ensor is recommended, as discussed fully by Zbinden (see

Selective Bibliography). The LD_{50} of each of the single components is determined. If the toxicities of the two components are strictly additive, the LD_{50} of any combination should be clearly predictable when plotted on a coordinate system. Two medicines are considered to induce more than additive acute toxicity if the combined LD_{50} is clearly greater than the plotted sums of the LD_{50} of each. If the opposite trend is demonstrated for their combined LD_{50}s, this may be taken as evidence of mutual antagonism.

(ii) Subacute toxicity studies. Toxicity studies of 30 to 90 days are demanded by many regulatory authorities for the evaluation of fixed-ratio combination medicines. They are conducted in different animals (most commonly rats and dogs) with at least three different dosages.

The selection of dosage ratio is the most difficult decision in practice. Because of marked differences between biological half-lives of medicines in animals and man the testing of a combination in an experimental animal will often lead to ratios of blood and tissue levels which are vastly different from those obtained in man given the same mixture of active substances. Adjustment of the dose ratio for each species according to the pharmacokinetics of the components is extremely difficult and requires considerable information on pharmacokinetics in animals and man. Furthermore, in each species, differences in degrees of induction of drug-metabolising ezymes and competition for excretory mechanisms are to be expected, and these factors may also be influenced by dosage. Not more than a fraction of the various combinations of medicines which might be administered to a patient can possibly be thoroughly evaluated experimentally for interactions.

5.3.3. Biochemical and in vitro studies

Drug interactions cannot readily be predicted without accurate knowledge of the mechanisms of the actions of the medicines concerned. Extrapolation of knowledge from biochemical pharmacology to clinical medicine has to be done with an appreciation of the difficulties in the application of fundamental biochemical principles to medical practice. Yet this is necessary if the hazards of interactions during drug therapy are to be anticipated and possible advantageous interactions exploited.

For absolute predictability all the receptor sites to which the medicine and the interacting agent relate would have to be identified, the physiological consequences determined, and the concentrations and degree of persistence of both medicine and interactor at these receptor sites defined. The limitations in attaining this degree of information often result in our present incomplete understanding of such fundamental processes as the molecular binding of medicines, the rate of formation and the nature of metabolites produced by enzymes during biotransformation, or the results of reaction in the body with other chemicals. When available, information of this type is chiefly derived from experimental animals, and there are uncertainties in extrapolation to humans.

Reference has already been made to the common and fallacious tendency to ascribe an interaction between two medicines to a single mechanism, whereas often drug-drug interactions may occur at several biochemical points. Even prediction of an interaction between similar pharmacological agents may be inaccurate. In vitro studies may be of value in evaluating redistributional drug-drug interactions, and these will be discussed in further detail later.

5.4. Clinical guidelines

Astute observation by clinicians is invaluable in detecting adverse drug-drug interactions in man. The reasons for this are twofold: first, many of the described interactions resulting from in vitro or from animal experimentation are not observed in humans and therefore have little relevance in clinical practice; secondly, reports of drug interactions in man based upon single case descriptions, studies of normal volunteers, or small numbers of patients under control conditions do not necessarily reflect the true situation in practice. In order to assess the significance and importance of drug interactions it is necessary to obtain clinical evidence of the existence of the interaction, its frequency of occurrence, and the consequences of the event for patients. Unfortunately, there is a paucity of data of this nature.

Adverse drug interactions in man are best identified by intensive monitoring, which is described further in Chapter 6.

5.4.1. Classification

Drug-drug interactions can be assigned to one of three categories of clinical significance:

(i) Major clinical significance. This includes those interactions which are well documented and which have the potential of being harmful to the patient.

(ii) Moderate clinical significance. This includes those interactions for which more documentation is needed for their real implications to be appreciated, and/or it has been established that the potential harm to the patient is less than in the first category.

(iii) Minor clinical significance. This includes those interactions which are of least significance for one or more of the following reasons: documentation is poor; the potential harm to the patient is slight; or the incidence of the interaction is low.

5.4.2. Individual variations in response

Because of differences in genetic constitution, age, underlying disease, renal and hepatic status, environmental influences, and end-organ responses, mode of administration of the medicine concerned, and other factors, it frequently happens that the specific conditions under which two interacting medicines are administered are most important in determining the outcome of an interaction. In particular individuals an interaction of major potential importance may produce no ill effects at all, while another interaction which might be assigned to the category of minor clinical significance may result in a dangerous and even life-threatening situation. Thus, the unique circumstances of the individual patient need always to be kept in mind when the clinical significance of drug interactions is considered. It is for this reason that preclinical and in vitro prediction of drug interactions are of such strictly limited value in practice.

The variables associated with drug-drug interactions fall into two major groups: patient factors (including disease states, genetic factors, age and environmental factors), and drug administration factors:

(i) Disease states. Patients with certain diseases may respond differently to medicines and to combinations of medicines than patients not so affected. Certain illnesses may predispose a patient to, or protect him from, the adverse effects of a drug interaction.

Renal disease associated with a fall in glomerular filtration rate and/or impairment of renal tubular function may result in impaired clearance and consequent increase in plasma levels of medicines. An alteration in volume of distribution of a medicine in patients with renal failure may have a similar effect. In such circumstances the likelihood of adverse drug interactions may be correspondingly increased. Likewise, alterations in plasma proteins and modifications in drug-plasma protein binding associated with renal disease may predispose patients to drug interactions.

Theoretically, impairment of hepatic function may affect drug metabolism and detoxification, resulting in increased blood levels and altering the probability of interactions. Hypoalbuminaemia may modify the severity of interactions involving the displacement of medicines from protein-binding sites. These latter examples appear to be less important in practice.

(ii) Genetic factors. The genetic constitution of an individual may have an important influence on disposition of medicines. In certain cases genetic effects on the pharmacokinetics of a medicine are clearly defined; however, more often it is not possible to predict from simple genetic considerations which patients are likely to be adversely disposed or otherwise to a particular medicine or drug interaction. Both monogenically and polygenically transmitted traits may predispose to adverse drug effects. Large interindividual differences in rates of elimination of many commonly used medicines exist, and these are mainly under genetic control. Evidence for this derives from family and twin studies. An important source of drug toxicity is accumulation in the body, due to the fact that interindividual differences are not sufficiently taken into account in adjusting dosage. Differences in the degree of induction of drug metabolism by enzymes also appear to be under genetic control. On the other hand, interindividual differences in the extent of inhibition of drug metabolism appear to be influenced more by environmental than genetic factors.

(iii) Environmental factors can significantly modify patients' drug biotransforming capacity. For example, large-scale environmental exposure to agents such as insecticides, nicotine, 3-4 benzpyrene and caffeine, or chronic administration of certain medicines either alone or in combination can influence the duration and intensity of drug action. These and other environmental effects may modify drug disposition at several possible different sites, including absorption, biotransformation, receptor interaction and elimination. Drug interactions at more than one site may occur simultaneously, resulting in either synergistic or antagonistic effects. (These multiple potential sources of environmental influence on the predominantly genetic control of variations in drug disposition suggest only limited clinical application of genetic studies in evaluating and predicting drug interactions. However, several investigators believe that genetic factors may regulate the extent to which various environmental factors alter drug-metabolising capacity, and that drug metabolism in a particular individual may be a more uniform process than previously suspected even for chemically unrelated drugs.)

(iv) Age. Adverse psychiatric incidents in elderly patients treated with psychotropic medicines are disturbingly common. Reference has already been made to the undesirable degree of sedation, confusion, disorientation, disinhibition reactions, and aggressive outbursts that can develop in old patients who receive such therapy. Taking into account the vulnerability of the elderly brain to such agents, it is little wonder that combination drug therapy regularly causes adverse mental and psychiatric effects.

There is some evidence that the responses of the young child's brain to certain medicines may differ from responses in adults. For example, phenobarbitone may, paradoxically, cause excitation in young children, and amphetamine and amphetamine-like substances may have different actions on the brains of young, disturbed children with hyperkinetic and aggressive disruptive behaviour syndromes to their actions on the brains of normal children and adults.

(v) Drug administration factors. Numerous factors relating to the administration of medicines concerned in interactions might modify the expression of adverse effects. These include:

> (a) Sequence of administration (the order in which two interacting medicines are taken may modify the clinical outcome);
> (b) Route of administration (some interactions only occur when both medicines are given orally; other interactions may be more severe when one or both are given by the parenteral route);
> (c) Time of administration (certain interactions are

more likely to be important when the time period between administration of the interacting medicines is short);

(d) Duration of therapy (some period of concomitant administration may be necessary and may vary from hours to weeks);

(e) Dosage (in general, adverse drug interactions are more likely to assume clinically significant proportions when large doses of one or both medicines are given).

5.4.3. *Redistributional drug interactions*

When it is suspected that a drug-drug interaction results from the displacement of one medicine from plasma-protein-binding sites by another (the interactor), it is necessary to establish the following before such an association can be proven:

(i) That the medicine is displaced by the interactor from human plasma proteins in vitro;

(ii) That the interaction results in a rise in free drug in the plasma in vivo, together with a fall in total plasma concentration of the displaced drug;

(iii) That redistribution can wholly account for the observed pharmacological effects. Useful indicators are the observation of a rapid and relatively short-lived onset of enhanced pharmacological activity and the reproduction of the effect by another chemically similar displacer.

The main interactions in which redistribution is believed to be a primary mechanism involve the oral anticoagulants and the oral hypoglycaemic agents. Much higher standards of proof are required than are at present generally provided before redistributional mechanisms can be given the pre-eminent position they currently hold in the literature.

5.5. Fixed-ratio combinations

When two or more active principles are combined in a fixed dose, the combination is treated for regulatory purposes as a new medicine and must be submitted to standard toxicity testing. Each of the active components and the combination are tested independently for safety. (In most cases, known medicines with well-documented pharmacological and toxicological backgrounds are selected for combinations.)

It may be deemed unnecessary to test a new combination when it comprises the same constituents, but in different proportions, as a medicine which has already been tested.

If a compound with well-known toxicity is included in a fixed drug combination, it is essential to determine whether the combination with another medicine modifies the toxicity of the first.

Detailed arguments for and against the use of fixed-dose combinations in clinical practice fall outside the scope of this book. In brief, such combinations may be warranted if they show clear evidence of efficacy and if each component makes a positive contribution to the therapeutic effect of the combination. Risks of adverse reactions should not be multiplied unless at the same time there is overriding benefit. Each component should be given at a dose level that may be expected to make optimal contribution to the total effect, taking into account considerations of safety in addition. There certainly are cases in which fixed-dose combinations meet all these requirements and may be regarded as valuable in drug therapy.

The overriding objection to many fixed-dose combinations is that they deny the physician flexibility to adjust the dosage of each medicine according to the patient's need, but the use of certain combinations is admissible on grounds of convenience for the patient, provided there is no risk of additional hazard.

5.5.1. Fixed-ratio combination medicines

Zbinden has recommended the following strategy for the testing of fixed-ratio combination medicines containing constituents which have already been approved by regulatory authorities, and are regarded as effective and safe in their own right:

(i) The theoretically possible interactions are identified, taking into account the pharmacological and toxicological properties of the active principles;

(ii) Animal experiments are designed to provide information as to whether the pharmacological and toxicological profiles of the active ingredients are modified when the components are administered together. Experiments are carried out to test the likelihood of predicted interactions occurring in test animals in doses corresponding to those used in man;

(iii) The available clinical experience of the pharmacological and toxic effects of each of the single components is considered;

(iv) Clinical studies are designed and previous case reports evaluated to determine whether the pharmacological and toxicological effects are significantly modified when the medicines are given in combination;

(v) The pharmacokinetic characteristics (absorption and elimination kinetics and distribution of single doses) of the active ingredients and of the combination are investigated in suitable animal experiments. Possible competition for protein binding sites may be investigated in vitro;

(vi) Steady-state blood levels of the active ingredients and the combination are determined in appropriate animal systems, using the route of administration anticipated to be used in man;

(vii) Bioavailability of the active ingredients is tested in man after single administration of the combination product;

(viii) Steady-state blood levels of the active ingredients and the pattern of the major metabolites in blood and urine are determined in man.

5.6. Potential interactions of single-entity medicines

Zbinden has suggested guidelines for the prediction of likely or possible drug-drug interactions in which a new single-entity medicine may be involved:

(i) Once the important pharmacological and toxicological properties of a new medicine have been identified, animal experiments are designed to assess the effects in combination with other compounds most likely to be used concurrently with the new entity. It has already been noted in this chapter that animal studies are of very limited value in the prediction of drug-drug interactions in clinical practice;

(ii) In early clinical trials the therapeutic and toxic effects of the new medicine are compared in patients with and without concomitant drug therapy. Again, the combinations studied are those which are likely to be used in practice. When evidence of adverse interference is found, further appropriate clinical pharmacological studies are initiated;

(iii) Pharmacokinetic studies of the new medicine in combination with another medicine are considered only when theoretical chemical reasons exist for their likely interaction (e.g. chelating properties, strong protein-binding characteristics, pH-dependent excretion, etc.) or when it is necessary to clarify unexplained changes of the pharmacological or toxicological profile of the medicine induced by concurrent use of a second medicine. The pharmacokinetic investigation should include blood level monitoring of the interacting medicine as well, when the blood level of the latter may be critical to its safety.

5.7. Summary and conclusions

(i) The possible relevant clinical results of a drug-drug interaction may be a beneficial effect, an adverse effect, or a diminution of efficacy. The majority of drug-drug interactions are not of any clinical consequence.

(ii) The commonest adverse effects of drug-drug interactions are cumulative toxicity with depression of the central nervous or cardiovascular systems.

(iii) The following medicines are most likely to be associated with drug-drug interactions: those with narrow therapeutic margins; acidic medicines with high degrees of plasma protein binding; medicines which transform enzymically to toxic metabolites.

(iv) Animal studies are of limited value in predicting adverse drug-drug interactions in humans.

(v) The clinical expressions of drug-drug interactions are frequently significantly influenced by interindividual variations in patient response, disease states, genetic factors, age, environmental factors and conditions of administration of the medicines concerned.

(vi) In the prediction of safety of a fixed-ratio combination of two medicines each of the active components is tested independently for safety, as well as the combination. The development of new fixed-ratio combinations is warranted only if each component makes a positive contribution to the efficacy of the combination.

Selective Bibliography

Council of Drugs of the American Medical Association (1970) Fixed-dose combinations of drugs. JAMA 213:1172

Hansten PD (1979) Drug interactions. Lea and Febiger, Philadelphia

Koch-Weser J, Sellars EM (1971) Drug interactions with coumarin anticoagulants. N Engl J Med 285:487 and 547 (2 parts)

MacGregor AG (1965) Review of points at which drugs can interact. Proc R Soc Med 58:943

Prescott LF (1969) Pharmacokinetic drug interactions. Lancet 1969 II:1239

Rawlins MD (1978) Drug interactions and anaesthesia. BR J Anaesth 50:689

World Health Organisation (1968) Principles for the clinical evaluation of drugs. WHO Tech Rep Ser 403

Zbinden G (1976) Drug combinations — Drug interactions. In: Zbinden G (ed) Progress in toxicology, vol 2. Springer, Berlin Heidelberg New York

6 Monitoring drug safety in clinical practice

6.1. Introduction

Over the past 10-15 years, society has become increasingly preoccupied with the safety of medicines. This reaction, commonly attributed simply to "thalidomide", reflects in fact a more widespread concern with the rights and protection of the consumer in every field and with ecology and the preservation of the environment. In the development of new medicines today the pharmaceutical industry spends vast amounts of time and money on the evaluation of safety before a human being is exposed to them. Furthermore, the demands of the public and of regulatory authorities, together with the stringent requirements for safety of industry and physicians alike, have tended to make efforts for the assurance of safety of a new medicine ever more rigorous.

Whereas heightened awareness and improved techniques in anticipating possible adverse effects of medicines are to be welcomed, it is equally important that the issues of drug safety are seen in perspective. No medicine can be regarded as entirely safe, and the therapeutic use of a medicine has to be regarded on the basis of a risk-benefit evaluation. This point is frequently not appreciated by the lay public or the mass media, nor occasionally even by drug regulatory authorities! The demand for completely safe medicines is naive. There is a danger that excessive preoccupation with preclinical evaluation of safety may make the cost of developing new medicines prohibitive. It is the pharmaceutical industry that is almost entirely responsible for the development of new medicines. It is essential that unnecessary disincentives to drug development should be removed as far as possible.

The difficulties in extrapolating and predicting human responses from animal studies have been referred to repeatedly in this book. The final test of safety of a new medicine can only be its record in clinical practice. If methods of evaluating safety in humans could be refined it might be possible to reduce the cost, duration and tedium of preclinical evaluation. However, earlier exposure of humans to potential risks from new medicines is always attended by important ethical considerations relating to the maximum possible protection of the individual. Herein lies one of the most important challenges to clinical pharmacology today.

6.2. The diagnosis of adverse drug reactions in practice

An adverse drug reaction (ADR) may be regarded as an unfavourable change in a patient's condition which is believed to be due to a medicine which is given in normal doses for an appropriate indication. This definition does not include drug poisoning. A clinically significant ADR normally results in a decrease of dosage or cessation of therapy, or requires special treatment, or suggests that future therapy with the medicine for the patient concerned or for other patients may carry a significant risk.

Adverse drug reactions fall broadly into one of two main categories:

(i) Adverse effects that might be anticipated from knowledge of the pharmacological action or actions of the medicines concerned. An individual patient may be particularly sensitive to pharmacological doses of a medicine or may experience an unwanted predictable action of a medicine related to its activity but not to its planned therapeutic effect;

(ii) Adverse effects that are unrelated to known pharmacological actions of the medicines. Such reactions may be a manifestation of allergic sensitisation to a medicine caused by previous exposure to the same medicine or to a chemically related substance mediated by an immune reaction, or of an idiosyncratic response which, as far as is known, does not have an immune basis. In certain instances idiosyncratic reactions may be genetically determined.

6.2.1. Criteria for a causal relationship

Real difficulties exist in practice in establishing a causal relationship between an adverse reaction and the aetiological agent (the medicine). In general, the criteria for causation of disease by an aetiological agent have been examined by clinicians and epidemiologists and the following principles, published by the Surgeon General's Advisory Committee on Smoking and Health (see Selective Bibliography), have received wide acceptance; they can logically be applied to the evaluation of adverse drug reactions:

(i) The association should be consistent, which implies that findings should be replicated when the association is studied in different localities and by different methods;

(ii) The association should be a strong one; this refers to both the magnitude of the association and the existence of a dose-response relationship;

(iii) The association should be specific or "distinctive". In a distinctive association the relationship between the suspected agent and the effect should be distinctive for those two entities. The likelihood of a particular disorder being associated with a specific aetiological agent is less if that disorder also frequently occurs in association with other conditions;

(iv) There should be a reasonable temporal relationship between exposure to the alleged cause and development of the alleged effect;

(v) The association should be coherent, i.e. it should be

plausible according to "known facts in the natural history and biology of the disease".

These criteria are valuable for the validation of causal relationships of adverse reactions and specific drugs. However, such validation may be particularly difficult to make in the field of drug therapy.

6.2.2. Difficulties in validating adverse drug reactions

The problems in establishing a causal relationship between an ADR and a medicine given in the course of an illness have been examined by Koch-Weser and by Karch and Lasagna (see Selective Bibliography).

Very few ADRs are clinical events unique to the medicine itself, nor do they usually present laboratory findings which differentiate them from the features of the patient's underlying illness. Many drug-treated patients with severe illnesses suffer during their clinical course unexpected and untoward events which may be attributable to the natural history or complications of the underlying disease. Such events may be confused with drug effects and vice versa. These difficulties are compounded by the fact that patients with serious illnesses (particularly those in hospital) often receive several medicines concomitantly. It is precisely these patients who are most susceptible to ADRs.

Problems also exist in the identification of less severe drug effects, such as nausea, vomiting, diarrhoea, constipation, skin rash, drug fever, and others. Here "background noise" may obscure real effects. These minor symptoms are no different to the recognised effects which may be noted during treatment with a placebo. (When placebo has been used in a trial as a control for an active medicine the side-effects tend to assume a similar form to the effects of the active medicine itself. This suggests that pre-existing conditions which might otherwise have gone unnoticed are uncovered and regarded as side-effects.) The incidence of placebo-related side-effects has varied in published reports from less than 1% to as much as 60%.

The most obvious approaches to confirming a drug aetiology for an adverse event are "dechallenge" and "rechallenge". With dechallenge an adverse drug effect may normally be expected to subside or disappear rapidly on discontinuation of therapy. Often this is not the case. Medicines or metabolites of medicines with a long duration of action and which persist in the body may continue to exert adverse effects long after treatment has been discontinued. Adverse effects which result from structural damage or immunological change of tissues do not readily revert to normal with removal of the primary stimulus.

Problems also exist with rechallenge. There are many false-positive and false-negative responses in clinical studies involving rechallenge. At the time of rechallenge the set of circumstances predisposing to the development of the original reaction may not be present. Furthermore, ethical problems exist in rechallenging a patient with a medicine to which he or she has already reacted unfavourably. Repeat exposure to a medicine which has induced a skin rash, hepatitis, bronchial constriction or anaphylaxis may have serious and possibly fatal results. Rechallenge studies are probably only justified when it is of vital importance to the patient that the relationship between an adverse reaction and a medicine be established beyond doubt. Repeated use of the medicine concerned would then be regarded as life-saving.

Not uncommonly the temporal relationship between medicine and adverse effect is not easily demonstrable. Certain complications of drug therapy may occur in a silent form and not be immediately apparent, therefore they may not be readily associated with their true cause. On the other hand, underlying diseases may be present although silent at the time of onset of therapy. Gall-stones, carcinoma, and thrombosis are examples of conditions which may have been silent at the outset of therapy and which may later declare themselves falsely as apparent complications of treatment.

There are great difficulties in confirming adverse reactions to medicines in the laboratory. No specific laboratory tests exist which can reliably detect or confirm drug sensitivity. For example, in vitro laboratory evaluation of lymphocyte activation in response to antigenic stimulation by a medicine suspected of being a sensitising agent has often been considered. Numerous published papers have claimed a close correlation between clinical hypersensitivity and the in vitro response of the patient's lymphocytes to the medicine. Other workers have failed to find such a correlation. The difficulties in interpretation exist in the large number of false-positive and false-negative reactions. Those medicines which cause adverse effects only after they have been metabolised in vivo will not show evidence of toxicity in vitro. Moreover, those adverse reactions that are critically dependent upon dose may not be simulated in the laboratory unless diligent attention is given to dose-response relationships.

6.3. Physicians' evaluations of adverse drug reactions

The inherent difficulties in diagnosing and confirming adverse drug reactions inevitably result in a wide lack of concordance in physicians' opinions as to what constitutes an ADR. The physician is particularly handicapped in perceiving associations between medicines and adverse events which do not fall within his or her concepts of the scope of effects of the medicine concerned. The Boston Collaborative Drug Surveillance Programme group quotes the example of the unexpected association of acute gastrointestinal bleeding and intravenously administered ethacrynic acid. The association of that complication was found to be 26% in 105 patients, yet in no instance had the physician attributed the bleeding to the medicine. (Routine computer analysis of total data had readily demonstrated this association.)

Even clinical pharmacologists whose particular functions include the diagnosis and detection of adverse drug reactions achieve a low concordance rate. Evaluators tend to have definite patterns of judgement, attributable to subconscious preconceptions.

New Zealand general practitioners varied widely in what they considered constituted an ADR. The medical experience and the particular interests of the doctor are very important in the final appreciation of an ADR. Concordance amongst general practitioners was greater when a serious and well-known drug reaction was noted.

It is likely that the recognition of entirely novel adverse effects is always going to be difficult. At the same time, physicians' reports will always constitute an important source of information about untoward effects caused by medicines. Only practising physicians observe a population at risk which is sufficiently large to reveal many of the reactions to commonly used medicines.

Reporting of cause-effect relationships could be improved by definition of the degree of certainty with which the observer makes the association. Karch and Lasagna have stressed this, and they have proposed the following qualification of relationships:

(i) Definite. A reaction that follows a temporal sequence from administration of the medicine, or in which a toxic drug level has been established in body fluids or tissues; that follows a known response pattern to the suspected medicine, and that is confirmed by improvement on stopping the medicine and by reappearance of the reaction on repeated exposure. (Reservations as to dechallenge and rechallenge studies were referred to in Section 6.2.2).

(ii) Probable. A reaction that follows a temporal sequence from administration of the medicine, that follows a known response pattern to the suspected medicine, that is confirmed by dechallenge, and that could not be explained by known characteristics of the patient's condition.

(iii) *Possible.* A reaction that follows a reasonable temporal sequence from administration of the medicine, that follows a known response pattern to the suspected medicine, and that could have been caused by the patient's clinical state, or other forms of therapy administered to the patient.

(iv) *Conditional.* A reaction that follows a reasonable temporal sequence from administration of the medicine, but does not follow a known response pattern to the suspected medicine, and yet cannot be explained by the patient's clinical state.

The function of this last category is to retain temporarily those cases that may be manifesting an undescribed adverse drug reaction and to allow later reclassification when more information becomes available. This category helps to prevent the loss of previously unsuspected drug reactions and to identify new ones.

(v) *Doubtful.* Any suspected reaction that does not meet the criteria above.

Evaluation of ADRs based on definite and probable reactions tends to underestimate the true incidence of adverse reactions, while findings that include possible reactions tend to overestimate the incidence.

6.4. Reporting and monitoring adverse drug reactions

The evaluation of safety of a medicine once it is in general use in the community is in its infancy in many countries. Development in this field of drug safety could increase the confidence of drug regulatory authorities, the lay public, and the producers of medicines (although it could be argued that the lay public will never be able to accept this method of safety evaluation). It could serve to shorten the preclinical evaluation process, with a saving in money as well as time, and possible alleviation of the present disincentives to the development of new medicines. Important new medicines should reach patients with the minimum of delay.

All systems of evaluating adverse drug reactions should detect one or more of the following:

(i) A sudden increase in reporting of a particular adverse effect;

(ii) A gradual increase or a particular trend in reporting of an adverse effect;

(iii) An increase in reporting of an adverse effect of particular interest, even if its incidence is small;

(iv) Adverse drug reactions which are of value in studying pharmacological mechanisms.

In the implementation of surveillance programmes a balance has to be struck so that the inclusion of excessive detail is avoided. Such detail reduces the relevance of essential data. Consideration has to be given not only to relevance but also to the cost and accuracy with which it can be acquired. Standards of data collection should be uniform as far as is possible. An ideal surveillance programme might also provide for the evaluation of efficacy. For example, the Boston programme has attempted to provide information about drug utilisation, as well as adverse effects, which has included the following: the extent of drug use; the relative frequencies of various indications; the degree of utilisation of individual medicines; and the variability of utilisation patterns according to hospital and geographical area.

In considering detailed methods of investigation it should be pointed out that no single approach offers a comprehensive system for the recognition of unwanted drug effects with a minimum of delay.

6.4.1. Voluntary reporting

For as long as doctors have been using medicines this method of reporting of adverse effects has been in operation. Physicians frequently sound the earliest warnings of problems associated with medicines, and they serve to alert regulatory authorities. A system which depends upon voluntary reporting of adverse effects can be developed to elevate standards of therapy and to maintain a high level of awareness amongst physicians.

No definite information exists as to how effective voluntary reporting systems are, or to what extent the incidence of iatrogenic disease they appear to reflect is real. There is little way of determining the accuracy of reports, and it is impossible to determine within wide limits the incidence of reported reactions amongst patients taking a particular medicine. Comparison with other patients or with the normal population may not be possible. Sometimes additional methods of investigation are required before a suspected reaction can be confirmed, or a medicine can be exculpated. These special tests cannot normally be implemented within a voluntary reporting system. So much depends upon physicians suspecting a particular association. A further difficulty is that voluntary reporting tends to be active-ingredient-based and not product-based, so that often important potential information is lost.

Where mandatory or compulsory notification of adverse drug reactions has been implemented (for example, in Sweden), there have been problems of overemphasis and overreporting. It is important to maintain freedom of reporting and to avoid an authoritarian approach. In any event, controlled reporting can only be implemented in those countries where the population is comparatively small and either prescriptions and hospital discharge diagnoses are prepared for purposes of accounting in national computer files or medical record linkage is in operation. Such systems have involved considerable expense and have tended to produce enormous volumes of data lacking in uniformity of expression and terminology. They have been further limited by incompleteness of records, and by omission of details which may be essential for an appreciation of adverse drug reactions.

6.4.2. Intensive case-orientated hospital reporting

The best documented example of intensive case-orientated hospital reporting of adverse drug reactions is the Boston Collaborative Drug Surveillance Programme. The function of this multi-hospital, international approach has been to record data of the everyday routine of clinical practice, without interfering in any way with the physician's freedom to apply what he or she considers to be optimum treatment.

The Boston survey has provided an opportunity to explore and detect the relevance of factors such as type of illness, duration of treatment and interaction with other drugs. The programme has shown that it is possible to evaluate efficacy as well as safety of medicines that are used in the hospital in-patient setting. An important claim made by the Boston group is that as a result of their activities the quality and quantity of spontaneous reporting of drug reactions has improved at the hospitals where they have functioned. They attribute their success in achieving an educational influence to several factors: a definition of adverse reactions which was easily applicable and operationally meaningful and which excluded trivial side-effects of drug therapy; feedback reports which made it clear to physicians that their opinions were being carefully observed and evaluated; and on-going emphasis on adverse drug reactions which probably increased the index of suspicion and focused attention on this problem throughout the hospitals concerned.

At the same time there are several limitations to the methods used by the Boston investigators. Inevitably, their system makes it difficult to provide for maximum accuracy of observation. Patient selection, dosage, and duration of therapy are not controlled. The most important shortcoming is that the data derived from studies of hospital-based patient populations have only limited application to non-hospital clinical practice.

The problems of determining the frequency of disease from hospital patients alone were analysed many years ago by

Berkson. Berkson suggested that there is inherent bias involved in evaluating disease incidence in the hospital compared with the whole population served by the hospital. This bias is believed to be based on the fact that patients with co-morbidity presentations are more likely to be admitted to hospital. Therefore, any hospital group which serves as a control does not correspond with what would be regarded as a control group in a non-hospitalised series of patients.

Other important reservations concerning hospital reporting of ADRs are the considerable expense involved in mounting and sustaining such programmes, the limited number of patients that can be evaluated in such a way, and the comparatively short duration of observation to which patients are subjected. Such surveillance systems are unlikely to identify rare reactions such as aplastic anaemia following chloramphenicol therapy, or reactions which result from long-term drug exposure such as interference with growth and development in children.

Out-patient drug surveillance schemes may go some way to meet certain limitations of in-patient studies. Long-term users of medicines can be followed in this way and the quantitation of relatively common serious effects of long-term therapy may be effectively carried out in a prospective out-patient study. On the other hand, drug events such as those occurring with a frequency of less than 1 in 5000 exposures cannot normally be detected with any form of prospective surveillance technique, and the study of transient mild drug effects in out-patients is not cost-effective taking into account the major logistic problems involved in conducting such a study. Finally, acute drug effects are more accurately and more economically studied within an in-patient setting.

6.4.3. Limited-release drug monitoring systems

There is a need for the study in detail of a cohort of recipients of new medicines in order to determine whether unsuspected adverse reactions which had been undetected in original clinical trials might be detectable after wider exposure. Limited-release drug monitoring of a new medicine offers the opportunities to record simple information on a larger selection of recipients.

Drug-monitoring studies promote interest amongst medical practitioners in therapeutics and in the appropriate and safe use of medicines. Monitored release may enable valuable data on the use of a medicine in clinical practice to be collected. On the other hand, in the absence of a suitable and appropriately randomised control group these studies cannot define the true spectrum and incidence of adverse drug effects, however large the cohort size may be. It is surprising how extensively a medicine can be used before its harmful effects are fully appreciated. Serious effects on the eye caused by chloroquine were not detected until 12 years after its introduction. Phenacetin was first introduced into medical practice in 1887, yet the first suspicions of the kidney damage which may be associated with its prolonged and excessive usage came only in 1953 — sixty-six years later. Even aspirin was widely used for many years before its potential for producing serious gastrointestinal bleeding was recognised. Limited-release studies are expensive to mount and they do not tend to develop new and original hypotheses. The cost in time and money to a company is not inconsiderable, and inevitably a monitored study adds to the cost of developing a new medicine. A further complication regarding limited release studies is that they may be construed as "promotional". This is likely to put restrictions upon the number of patients that may be studied. Such restrictions might reduce the amount of information likely to be gained from this approach.

6.4.4. Retrospective evaluation of drug safety
In retrospective, event-orientated case control studies the investigator begins by assembling people who are already diseased or non-diseased. From these "cases" and "controls"

the prevalence of previous exposure to the suspected aetiological agent is estimated. Patients are identified who have experienced a particular event. These patients are then compared with patients who had not experienced the event. The investigator has to determine the characteristics that differentiated the people under the study. Lenz used this method to show that thalidomide was the cause of epidemic phocomelia. The status of persons in the control and test groups as having or not having the target disease and in respect of their exposure or non-exposure to the aetiological agent has to be defined with accuracy. Since these matters are examined long after exposure or non-exposure, checking for accuracy may pose a particular problem.

On the positive side, this method of retrospective evaluation is comparatively inexpensive and has contributed much to knowledge about disease and pharmacology. The special advantages of such an event-orientated approach to drug safety are logistic. Compared with prospective studies they require a far smaller number of individuals to be studied. These advantages increase with the rarity of the condition under surveillance, particularly when the association with the suspected cause is strong, and when there is unlikely to be serious bias owing to differential failure of recall. In prospective studies exposures to environmental conditions may change. Such variables can more easily be taken into account in retrospective studies.

The retrospective study is not suitable for evaluation of efficacy of therapy or prophylaxis of disease, for which clinical trials have always to be done. It is also less appropriate than other methods for the study of conditions of high incidence and short duration.

There are several sources of error in retrospective studies:
(i) The choice of controls is potentially the most problematic. Members of the control group chosen for retrospective studies are not controls in the usual sense: they represent people who are non-diseased or unaffected by a particular

event, rather than people who have not been exposed. The retrospective selection of controls from hospitalised patients may introduce particular forms of bias. Ideally two kinds of controls should be studied — a population control group and a series of patients. Consistency in the frequency of the attributes of interest between the two control groups will strengthen confidence in the findings, and inconsistency will warn of possible biased selection.

(ii) Problems are also caused by simple memory failure or biased recollection. Patients who have experienced a particular adverse event are more likely to recall an association than those who have not experienced the event. Interviewers may unintentionally elicit positive information more assiduously from patients than from controls. This risk may be reduced by "blind" questioning, i.e. by keeping the interviewers ignorant of either the hypothesis that is being tested or the classification of the subjects, or both.

(iii) There is a hazard that in retrospective evaluation aetiological significance may be erroneously attached to attributes that are really the outcome of the disease itself.

It is rare that the findings deriving from retrospective studies have been shown to be wrong or in conflict with those of prospective studies, although the opportunities for this kind of comparison have been few.

6.5. Risk-benefit evaluations

The practising physician has to decide whether the risks of drug therapy to the patient are outweighed by the potential benefit. The quality of such a decision is highest when information concerning both aspects is as clear as possible. The physician takes into account the severity of illness of the patient, and the alternative treatments available. Individual physicians will always differ in their evaluations, and so will regulatory authorities. Furthermore, the relationships between efficacy and safety of a particular medicine will always be changing as new knowledge concerning either or both becomes available. There are times when developments in knowledge concerning efficacy or safety demand reassessment of the accepted place of a medicine in therapeutics. This represents an important aspect of therapeutics, where the consideration of safety represents only one side of the coin.

6.6. Summary and conclusions

(i) The surest criterion of safety of a medicine is its record of administration to humans. Improvement of methods of evaluation of safety of medicines in clinical practice is of fundamental importance.

(ii) The difficulties in establishing a causal relationship between a medicine and an adverse reaction attributable to it are compounded by the lack of clear-cut characteristics of adverse drug-induced events distinguishing them from features of an underlying illness or its complications. Moreover, laboratory tests that can reliably confirm drug toxicity do not exist.

(iii) A lack of concordance frequently exists in doctors' evaluation of adverse drug reactions. Improvement in this regard will require development and acceptance of rigorous criteria for the diagnosis of drug-induced diseases. Reports of adverse reactions are enhanced by qualification of the degree of certainty with which the observer has made the association: definite, probable, possible, conditional, or doubtful.

(iv) The strengths and limitations of prospective and retrospective drug surveillance programmes were examined. The potential value of well-designed and properly executed retrospective studies has probably been underestimated in the past.

(v) A risk-benefit assessment has to be made by the physician in prescribing any medicine. It is a challenge to all concerned that the physician is fully informed as to both sides of that equation.

Selective Bibliography

Colombo F, Shapiro S, Slone D, Tognoni G (eds) (1977) Epidemiological evaluation of drugs. Elsevier/North Holland, Amsterdam

Feinstein AR (1974) The biostatistical problems of pharmaceutical surveillance. Clin Pharmacol Ther 15:110

Finney DF (1965) The design and logic of a monitor of drug use. J Chronic Dis 18:77

Jick H (1977) The discovery of drug-induced illness. N Engl J Med 296:481

Karch FE, Lasagna L (1976) Evaluating adverse drug reactions. Adverse Drug Reaction Bulletin 59:204

Koch-Weser J, Sidel VW, Sweet RH, Kanarek P, Eaton AE (1969) Factors determining physician reporting of adverse drug reactions. N Engl J Med 280:20

Roberts RS, Spitzer WO, Delmore T, Sackett DL (1978) An empirical demonstration of Berkson's bias. J Chronic Dis 31:119-128

Sartwell PE (1974) Retrospective studies. Ann Intern Med 81:381

Surgeon General's Advisory Committee on Smoking and Health (1964) Smoking and health. United States Department of Health, Education and Welfare, Public Health Service Publication No.1103

Wilson AB (1977) Post-marketing surveillance of adverse reactions to new medicines. Br Med J 2:1001

Subject Index

"absolute safety" 13
abstinence syndrome 31
adverse drug reaction 84, 88, 89
aflatoxin B_1 51
aflatoxins 52
age, and drug responses 8
alcohol, see ethyl alcohol
alkylating agents 24, 52, 53
amphetamine 30, 34, 36, 67, 77
anaesthetics 24
analgesics 17, 66, 68
androgenic hormones 23, 24
animal studies 1
animal models of drug dependence 43, 44, 45
anorexiants 24, 37, 42
antacids 17
antibiotics 24
anticoagulants, oral 10, 66, 68, 69, 78
anticonvulsants 23, 24
antidepressants 65, 68
antiemetics 17
antihistamines 17, 23, 65
antihypertensive drugs 68
anti-inflammatory drugs 66, 67
antimalarial agents 24
antimitotic agents 51
antineoplastic agents 19, 23, 24
antituberculous agents 24
antitussives 17

arsenic 51, 53
atrioventricular conduction 65
atropine 8
atropine esterase 8

barbiturates 10, 24, 30, 32, 65, 67
behavioural abnormalities, drug-induced 20
belladonna alkaloids 10
benzodiazepines 38, 39
3-4 benzpyrene 76
beta-blockers 52, 65, 67
bias in evaluating disease 94
bioavailability 7
biotransformation status 9
blood-brain barrier 8
Boston collaborative drug surveillance programme 93
breast, malignant tumour of the female 21
busulphan 53

caffeine 10, 76
carcinogen, chemical 49
carcinogenicity testing 58
children 14
chlorambucil 53
chloramphenicol 53
chlornaphazin 53
creosote 53
coal tar 51, 53

co-carcinogens 53, 55
corticosteroids 53
contraceptives, oral 21, 63
coumarin anticoagulants 66, 67
cyclamates 53
cytotoxic agents 69

dechallenge studies 87, 89
DDT 4
dependence 29, 30
dialkyltriazines 51
diethyl stilboestrol 19
diethylene glycol 5
digitalis 67, 69
dimethylnitrosamine 52
diuretics 66, 67
dose-response 88
drug
— dependence 29
— -drug interactions 10, 63
— hypersensitivity 7
— surveillance 91, 94

electrophilic reactants 51
embryo, drug damage to 20
employees, clinical trials performed on 14
epidemiological patterns of drug dependence 41
ergot alkaloids 10
ethacrynic acid 88
ethyl alcohol 24, 30, 65

feticidal cannibalism 6
"first-hit" damage 6
fixed-ratio combination medicines 79, 80
fluoride 10, 13
folate antagonists 23, 24
formulation 5

gastrointestinal bleeding
— acute 10, 88
— chronic 10
genetic influences on drug action or toxicity 76, 85

glucuronidation systems 8
griseofulvin 53
growth retardation, drug-induced 20

heart block, drug-induced 65
husbandry, animal 8, 57
hypersensitivity reactions 10
hypnotics 66
hypoglycaemic agents 24, 66, 68, 69, 78

iatrogenic disease 92
idiosyncratic reactions 85
immunosuppressive agents 51, 53
insecticides 76
inter-species differences in drug responses and toxicity 7
intra-species differences in drug responses and toxicity 8
intraperitoneal administration of medicines 5
in vitro studies of carcinogenicity 59
iron preparations 17
iron dextran 53
isoniazid 10

laboratory diagnosis of ADRs 88
laxatives 17
lethal dose $_{50}$ (LD_{50}) 2, 71, 72
limited-release drug monitoring 94
lithium carbonate 24
local irritancy of medicines 7
LSD 24
lymphocyte stimulation 88

marihuana 24
melphalan 53
mercury, organic 23, 24
metabolite-mediated toxicity 12
methoxyflurane 13
methyl mercury 19
minerals 17
monitoring adverse drug reactors 90

Subject index

monoamine oxidase inhibitors 67
morphine 7, 30, 31, 67
moulds 52
mutagenicity studies 59

narcotic analgesics 24, 65, 67
nasal decongestants 17
nicotine 76
nitrogen mustards 53
nitrosamines 51, 53

oestrogens 51, 53
oral contraceptives 53
organic mercury 23, 24
over-the-counter preparations 17, 68

paracetamol 69
paternal sperm, drug effects 19
pentamethylphosphoramide 53
peptic ulceration, drug-induced 10
pharmaceutical industry 83, 84
phenobarbitone 77
phenols 53
phenothiazines 65
phenylbutazone 9, 53, 67
phocomelia, epidemic 96
placebo effects 86
porphyria 10
pregnancy, drug treatment 14
prisoners, drug treatment of 14
progesterone 53
prolonged toxicity studies 4
pronethalol 53
ß-propiolactone 53
psychomotor disorders, drug-induced 20
pyrolizidine alkaloids 52

quinidine 65, 67
quinine 24

radiomimetics 52
rechallenge studies 87

redistributional drug interactions 73, 78
reserpine 53
retrospective evaluation of drug safety 95
risk-benefit evaluation 83, 97

salicylates 10, 23, 24
sedatives 17, 66
sex hormones 24
single-dose studies 14
species differences in drug metabolism 3
spontaneous animal diseases 9
sulphonamides 5, 24
surface area, dose correction 11
sympathomimetic medicines 36, 37, 67, 68

tannic acid 53
teratogenesis 17
teratogenic zone 21
teratogens 24
thalidomide 17, 23, 24, 83, 96
— model 17
tolbutamide 67
tolerance 29, 34
toxicity studies
— acute 3
— prolonged 4, 5
tranquillisers 23, 24, 42
tretamine 53
tricyclic antidepressants 23, 24, 65, 67
tumours, drug-induced 55

urethan 52, 53

vagina, local toxicity 7
vaginal adenosis 19
— carcinoma 19
vitamins 17

warfarin sodium 23, 24

New Anticancer Drugs

Editors: S. K. Carter, Y. Sakurai

1980. 83 figures, 164 tables. XI, 220 pages
(Recent Results in Cancer Research,
Volume 70)
ISBN 3-540-09682-5

Quantitative Aspects of Risk Assessment in Chemical Cardiogenesis

Symposium held in Rome, Italy, April 3–6, 1979

Editors: J. Clemmesen, D. M. Conning, D. Henschler, F. Oesch
Technical Editing: A. Waring

1980. 64 figures, 56 tables. VII, 336 pages
(Archives of Toxicology, Supplement 3)
ISBN 3-540-09584-5

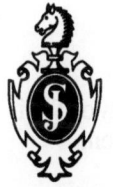

R. J. Tallarida, L. S. Jacob

The Dose-Response Relation in Pharmacology

1979. 108 figures, 26 tables. XIII, 207 pages
ISBN 3-540-90415-8

Springer-Verlag
Berlin
Heidelberg
New York

E. Gladike, H. M. v. Hattinberg

Pharmacokinetics

An Introduction

With contributions by W. Kübler,
W.-H. Wagner
Foreword by E. R. Garrett
Translated from the German by
P. J. Wilkinson

1979. 72 figures, 13 tables. IX, 141 pages
ISBN 3-540-09183-1

Carcinogenic Hormones

Editor: C. H. Lingeman

1979. 156 figures, 24 tables. XI, 196 pages
(Recent Results in Cancer Research,
Volume 66)
ISBN 3-540-08995-0

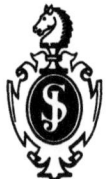

Toxicological Aspects of Food Safety

Proceedings of the European Society of Toxicology. Meeting held in Copenhagen,
June 19–22, 1977

Editor: B. J. Leonard

1978. 76 figures, 81 tables. XI, 392 pages
(Archives of Toxicology, Supplement 1)
ISBN 3-540-08646-3

Springer-Verlag
Berlin
Heidelberg
New York

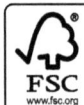

MIX
Papier aus verantwortungsvollen Quellen
Paper from responsible sources
FSC® C105338

If you have any concerns about our products,
you can contact us on
ProductSafety@springernature.com

In case Publisher is established outside the EU,
the EU authorized representative is:
**Springer Nature Customer Service Center GmbH
Europaplatz 3, 69115 Heidelberg, Germany**

Printed by Libri Plureos GmbH
in Hamburg, Germany